THE EASY AUTOIMMUNE PROTOCOL
COOKBOOK

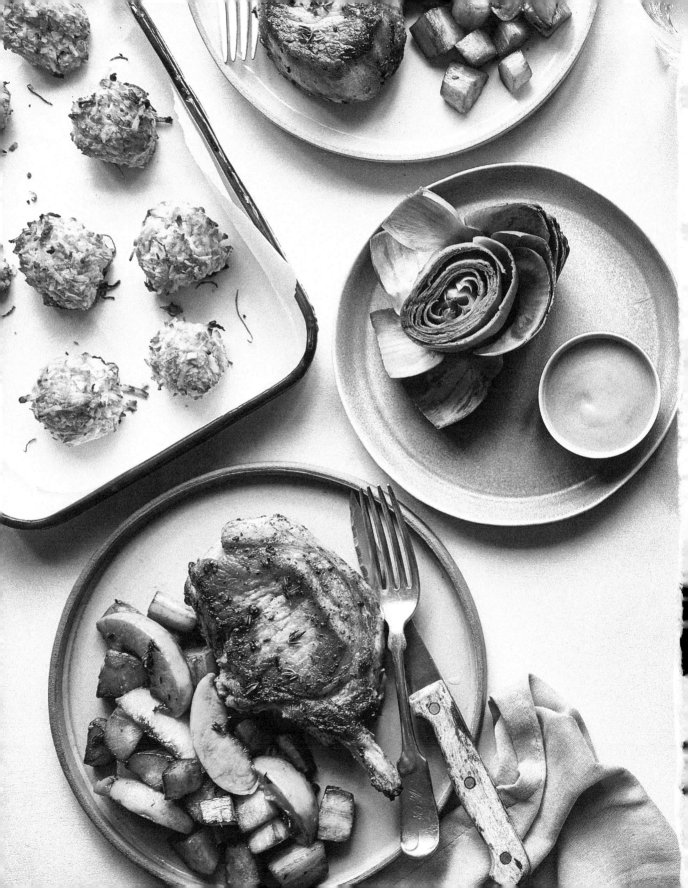

THE EASY AUTOIMMUNE PROTOCOL COOKBOOK

Nourish and Heal with 30-Minute, 5-Ingredient, and One-Pot Paleo Autoimmune Recipes

KARISSA LONG & KATIE AUSTIN

PHOTOGRAPHY BY **HÉLÈNE DUJARDIN**

ROCKRIDGE PRESS

For general information on our other products and services or to obtain technical support, please contact our Customer Care Department within the United States at (866) 744-2665, or outside the United States at (510) 253-0500.

Rockridge Press publishes its books in a variety of electronic and print formats. Some content that appears in print may not be available in electronic books, and vice versa.

Interior and Cover Designer: Linda Snorina

Art Producer: Hannah Dickerson

Editor: Rachelle Cihonski

Production Editor: Jenna Dutton

Photography © 2020 Hélène Dujardin, food styling by Anna Hampton

Decorative illustration courtesy of Vecteezy

Author photos courtesy of Alexandra Strimbu

Cover image: Grilled Chimichurri Shrimp and Cucumber Mint Salad, page 120

ISBN: Print 978-1-64611-867-0
       eBook 978-1-64611-868-7

R0

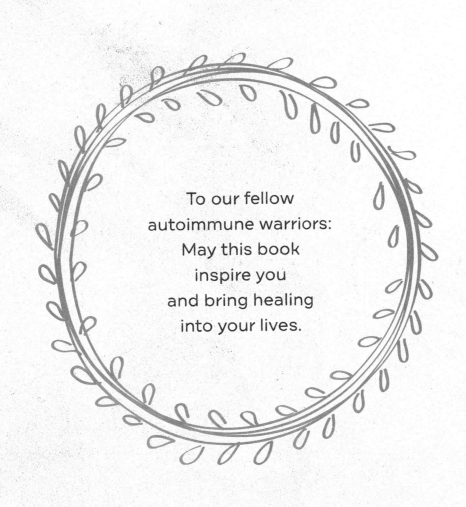

To our fellow
autoimmune warriors:
May this book
inspire you
and bring healing
into your lives.

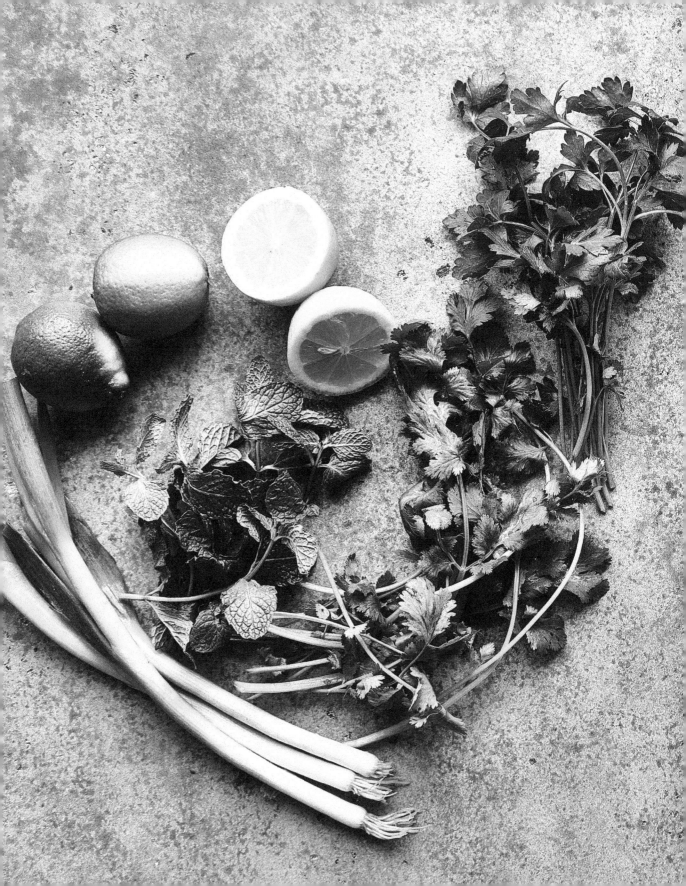

CONTENTS

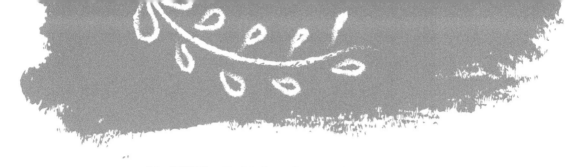

INTRODUCTION

Hello and welcome! We are so delighted that you have picked up this book and are taking your first (or next) step to healing your body using the power of diet and nutrition. That's right—you have the ability to improve your health by implementing strategies that are designed to nourish, regulate, and restore your well-being. Really, it's true!

We know it's possible because we have experienced it ourselves. Between the two of us, we have four autoimmune diseases—ulcerative colitis, Hashimoto's thyroiditis, postural orthostatic tachycardic syndrome, and ankylosing spondylitis—with symptoms ranging from fatigue, joint pain, heart palpitations, bleeding, and cramping to digestive distress. We lived with these symptoms for years, while our doctors continued to write us prescriptions for medicines designed to treat our symptoms but not heal the root cause.

It wasn't until we went on our own quest for answers that we truly began to understand the impact of food on our health. After poring over medical research and studying nutrition science, we found the autoimmune protocol, a way of eating intended to help people suffering from autoimmune diseases manage and reverse their symptoms. By successfully implementing the autoimmune protocol, we not only put our respective autoimmune diseases into remission, but we also healed our bodies and achieved optimal wellness. And if we can do it, so can you.

We created this book with the goal of making the autoimmune protocol simple, approachable, and straightforward. In the following chapters, we provide you with everything you need to be successful. In first chapter, we explain the background and science behind the protocol, detail the exact steps you should take to prepare, and provide a sample meal plan to get you started. In the rest of the book, we focus our attention all the wonderful dishes you can enjoy.

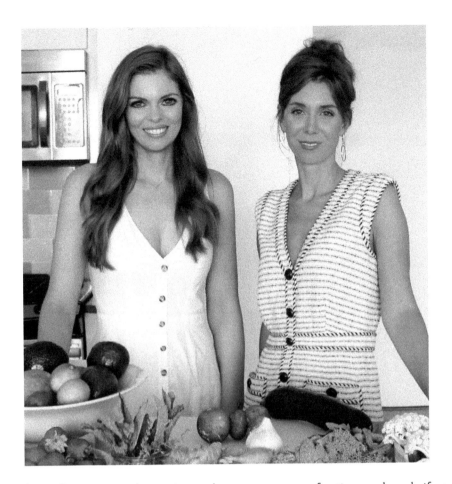

We know from personal experience that any new way of eating works only if you enjoy the foods you're eating, the recipes are easy to make, and you feel *satisfied*. In other words, the food you're making has to be delicious and satiating but also practical. So we are sharing with you more than 100 delicious recipes that check off all these criteria and also fit into the autoimmune protocol, meaning they are designed to nourish your body and regulate your immune system.

By the end of this book, there will be no more guesswork, intimidation, or frustration when it comes to the autoimmune protocol. Instead, you will be informed, organized, and, most important, motivated to embark on your own healing journey. We can't wait for you to get started and truly experience the power of this way of life.

XO,
Karissa & Katie

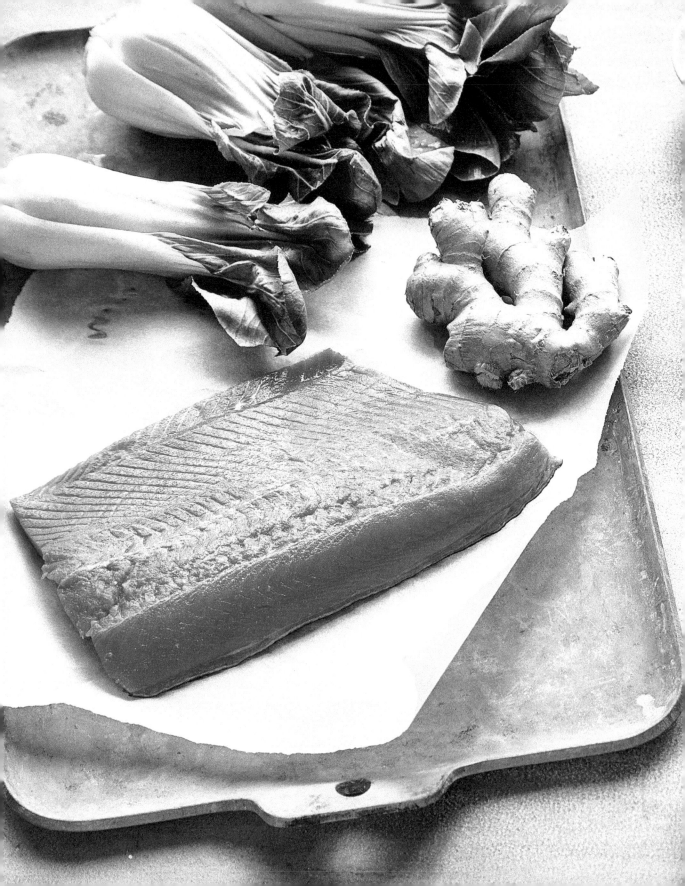

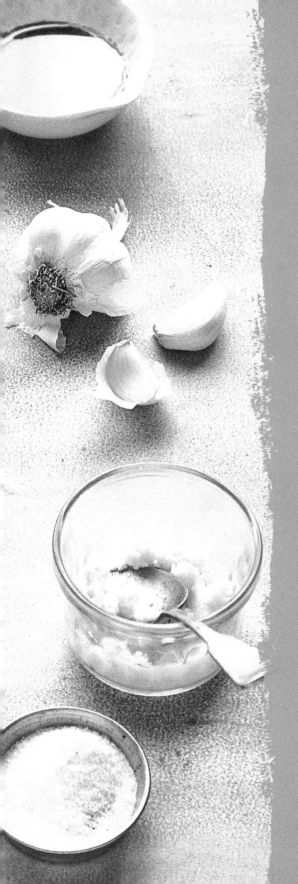

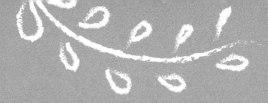

CHAPTER 1

AUTOIMMUNE DISEASE AND DIET

We know you can't wait to heal your body and are eager to get started on this wellness journey. But before you skip ahead to the recipes, we urge you to stop and take a few minutes to absorb all the information in this chapter. We firmly believe that knowledge is power, especially when it comes to your health. In the following pages, we are going to help you understand the science behind autoimmune disease, the role of your diet in both exacerbating and healing your symptoms, and how to easily set yourself up for success.

What Are Autoimmune Diseases?

Our bodies are equipped with a sophisticated defense system designed to protect us from harmful threats such as pathogens, toxins, parasites, bacteria, viruses, and other microbes. This intricate system is known as the immune system and is made up of several organs and thousands of cells that work collectively to fight off invaders and remove them from your body.

As long as your body's defense system is working properly, your immune system will go unnoticed. Problems arise when your immune system creates antibodies that end up attacking your own healthy cells and organs, not just the invaders. Essentially, your body's immune system can't tell the difference between healthy cells and invading cells, so it attacks what it was designed to protect. This leads to a variety of autoimmune diseases, depending on what organ or group of cells the immune system targets.

The Most Prevalent Autoimmune Diseases

The American Autoimmune Related Diseases Association defines autoimmune disease as a varied group of illnesses that affect almost every human organ system, including the nervous, gastrointestinal, and endocrine systems, as well as the eyes, skin, blood, and blood vessels. In all of the more than 100 autoimmune diseases that have been identified, the underlying problem is autoimmunity, which means the body's immune system becomes misdirected and attacks the organs it was designed to protect. Below are some of the most common autoimmune diseases.

Hashimoto's thyroiditis: Most prevalent in women, this condition is the result of the immune system attacking the thyroid. This can lead to hypothyroidism, where the thyroid does not make enough thyroid hormones. Symptoms can include (but are not limited to) weight gain and fatigue.

Inflammatory bowel disease (IBD): IBD is actually a group of diseases that includes Crohn's disease and ulcerative colitis, where the intestines become inflamed. The most common symptoms are cramping, diarrhea, and blood in the stool.

Lupus: This chronic condition can attack different parts of the body, including the skin, kidneys, nervous system, and brain. Symptoms vary but can include achy and swollen joints, fever, skin rashes, and fatigue.

Multiple sclerosis: This disease is the result of the immune system attacking and destroying the myelin coating, a fatty substance that protects the nerve cells. Symptoms include weakness, numbness, fatigue, tingling, and trouble walking or speaking.

Psoriasis: This condition is a direct result of the immune system attacking the skin cells so they become inflamed. Symptoms include skin rashes that are red and often covered with loose, silvery scales.

Rheumatoid arthritis: This condition results from inflammation in the joints that most commonly affects the hands, feet, wrists, elbows, knees, and ankles. Symptoms include swelling and pain in the joints.

What Causes Autoimmune Disease?

While there is not one specific trigger that causes people to develop these diseases, research has identified several common causes that contribute to autoimmunity.

Genetics: Genetics play a huge role in all aspects of your health, and this is particularly true for the functioning of your immune system. It is quite common for several members of a family to have the same autoimmune disease, as they share a similar genetic makeup. If you've already been diagnosed with one autoimmune disease, you are more likely to develop additional autoimmune diseases because you are genetically more predisposed to autoimmunity.

Diet: Your diet plays a significant role when it comes to developing an autoimmune disease. What you eat and drink (both the types of foods and the quality) can create conditions within your body that increase your risk for an autoimmune disease. These conditions include leaky gut (also known as permeability in your intestinal wall), increased and chronic inflammation, vitamin and nutrient deficiencies, and an overstimulated immune system.

Lifestyle: Factors such as chronic stress, poor sleep, and lack of movement all have the ability to increase your risk for autoimmune disease. Each of these factors, or a combination of them, can affect your body's immune function and contribute to developing autoimmune diseases.

Environment: Your body is constantly being exposed to chemicals, bacteria, pathogens, viruses, and other toxins within our environment. These toxins lurk in our homes in cleaning products, skincare items, and makeup, to name a few, and appear in our food as pesticides, herbicides, antibiotics, and genetically modified organisms (GMOs). They even exist in our water supply as chlorine, lead, and other chemicals. This regular exposure can trigger the development of autoimmune diseases.

Currently, there are no cures for autoimmune diseases. But the good news is that you can manage your disease and its symptoms—and sometimes even reverse them—by making some changes to your diet and lifestyle.

The Diet Connection

Your diet is an integral part of your health. This is especially true when you are suffering from an autoimmune disease. It's important to understand the link between autoimmune disease and diet so you can understand how powerful food can be for your well-being. The key to taking control of your diet and healing these conditions really comes down to two main principles.

1. AVOID FOODS THAT CONTRIBUTE TO LEAKY GUT AND INFLAMMATION

Processed foods: Most packaged and manufactured foods contain additives, artificial ingredients, preservatives, and sugars that put a strain on your immune system and promote chronic inflammation within the body.

Low-quality foods: Even the whole foods you are eating may be causing problems for your immune system. Conventional produce can contain pesticides, herbicides, and fertilizers. When it comes to protein, most meats and seafood are factory-farmed and come from animals are raised in conditions that are overcrowded and dirty (even fish!). To control disease, these animals are pumped full of antibiotics and other pesticides. All of these chemicals are passed on to us when we eat these foods, and our immune system is activated to attack these invaders.

WHAT DOES LEAKY GUT ACTUALLY MEAN?

"Leaky gut" plays a significant role in inflammation and autoimmunity. The walls of your intestines are designed to act as barriers in order to control what is absorbed into the bloodstream. They contain small gaps, called tight junctions, to allow the nutrients and water your body needs to pass through. When these tight junctions function properly, they also block the passage of harmful substances into the bloodstream. But when these tight junctions begin to fail, it creates permeability within the intestinal wall that allows toxins, bacteria, viruses, or undigested food particles to enter your bloodstream or lymphatic system. These foreign items are identified by your immune system, and it immediately springs into action. This constant activation causes inflammation in your body and can lead to autoimmune disease.

Leaky gut can be caused by several factors, including food sensitivities or allergies, an imbalance of gut flora (the organisms that naturally live in the gut), exposure to toxins, and chronic stress. Some common signs of a leaky gut are:

- Digestive issues such as chronic bloating, constipation, diarrhea, or stomach pain
- Skin issues such as acne, eczema, rashes, or rosacea
- Lack of energy or constant fatigue
- Headaches, brain fog, or mood imbalances
- Aching, swelling, or joint pain

If you are experiencing any of these symptoms or think you may have leaky gut, ask your doctor to test for it. Common leaky gut tests are the mannitol/lactulose test, parasite test, and bacteria dysbiosis test.

The good news is that a leaky gut can be treated and repaired. By addressing the factors that cause it (we'll tell you how later in this chapter), you can reseal your intestinal lining. In fact, many people find that by just addressing their leaky gut, some or all of their autoimmune symptoms subside.

2. LOAD UP ON NUTRIENT-DENSE FOODS

High-quality whole foods: Look for the following labels, which are found on foods that contain smaller amounts of chemicals and other toxins:

- **PROTEINS:** organic, grass-fed, grass-finished, heritage breed, pastured, wild-caught

- **FATS:** organic, unrefined, non-GMO

- **FRUITS AND VEGETABLES:** organic, non-GMO, local

Eat the rainbow: If you are suffering from an autoimmune disease, you most likely have some sort of micronutrient deficiency. That's why it is crucial to eat a wide variety of foods that are rich in nutrients and provide the vitamins and minerals your body needs to heal your gut and reduce inflammation. Here are some of the most vital nutrients and the foods that contain them:

- **VITAMIN A:** tuna, liver, carrots, sweet potatoes, cantaloupe

- **B VITAMINS:** beef, salmon, shellfish, poultry, organ meats, leafy greens

- **VITAMIN C:** oranges, grape-fruit, lemons, strawberries, broccoli, Brussels sprouts

- **VITAMIN D:** salmon, sardines, fish liver oil, mushrooms

- **VITAMIN E:** avocados, spinach, Swiss chard, butternut squash

- **CALCIUM:** leafy greens, figs, sardines

- **IRON:** liver, red meat, poultry, shellfish, leafy greens

- **MAGNESIUM:** avocados, salmon, halibut, bananas, leafy greens

- **POTASSIUM:** avocados, sweet potatoes, spinach, watermelon

- **ZINC:** shellfish, red meat, leafy greens

GUT-HEALING SUPERSTARS

Now that you know what an important role the gut plays in autoimmunity, you understand why it's important to eat foods that promote gut health and are extremely nutrient-dense. For ultimate healing, we recommend that you eat these foods regularly.

BONE BROTH: Rich in collagen, gelatin, and essential minerals, bone broth is the gold standard for gut-healing foods. You can make your own (Chicken Bone Broth, page 190, or Beef Bone Broth, page 191) or buy it at your local grocery store. Make sure you are buying bone broth, not stock or regular broth. Our favorite brands are Bonafide Provisions and Kettle & Fire.

GELATIN OR COLLAGEN FROM GRASS-FED SOURCES: Both come in powder form and are full of amino acids that help support the health of your body's connective tissue and heal your gut. Our favorite brands are Vital Proteins and Great Lakes.

FERMENTED VEGETABLES (SUCH AS SAUERKRAUT OR KIMCHI): The fermentation process produces healthy bacteria and enzymes that work to promote healthy gut flora. We like making our own versions, or you can buy fermented veggies. Look for them in the refrigerated section in the supermarket, and check the label to make sure the only ingredients, other than vegetables, are water and salt.

COCONUT YOGURT: Full of probiotics and healthy fats that aid in immune function, coconut yogurt is a staple in our kitchens. While we love making our own, homemade coconut yogurt is a lengthy process, so for this book and the recipes to come, we recommend buying it. Just make sure the only ingredients are coconut, water, and probiotic cultures. We like the brands Anita's and GT's CocoYo.

PROBIOTIC DRINKS (SUCH AS KEFIR OR KOMBUCHA): These fermented drinks are made from starter cultures and are full of probiotics that help rebalance the bacteria in your gut. Make sure to look for the flavors with the least amount of sugar. We like GT's Organic & Raw Kombucha and Kevita Kombucha.

Why the Autoimmune Protocol Works

The autoimmune protocol works because it focuses on healing your body from the inside out by taming inflammation and repairing your gut lining.

Inflammation is always present in your body. Some is advantageous—for instance, your body uses inflammation to heal when you get a scrape or a bruise. However, chronic inflammation can become a problem, especially when it causes overactivation of the immune system.

The foods you eat can promote inflammation. First off, many of the foods available to us on a modern diet contain toxins in the form of additives, artificial ingredients, preservatives, and sugars that cause inflammation within the body. This constant stream of processed foods puts a strain on our bodies and overstimulates our immune system. In addition, every person reacts differently to the foods they are eating and digesting. If your body is allergic, intolerant, or sensitive to foods you're eating, this could lead to inflammation.

When you remove these inflammatory foods from your diet and replace them with nourishing, nutrient-dense foods—as you will on the autoimmune protocol—you give your body an opportunity to heal. Inflammation in your body subsides and your gut lining begins to repair itself. The combination of reduced inflammation and a healed gut is the key to reducing or eliminating your autoimmune disease symptoms.

How the Autoimmune Protocol Works

What exactly is the autoimmune protocol (AIP)? In simple terms, AIP calls for you to temporarily eliminate all foods that are commonly found to be problematic for people with an autoimmune disease—in other words, the foods that are known to cause inflammation or leaky gut.

After you have seen significant improvements in your symptoms and reestablish a good health baseline, you can then slowly reintroduce foods into your diet. This reintroduction phase enables you learn what foods your body can tolerate and uncover which ones your body is sensitive to. By the end of the protocol, you will have created a customized long-term solution that works for you.

The Elimination Phase

During the elimination phase, you will remove from your diet categories of foods that are known to be problematic, along with all artificial ingredients, sweeteners, and processed foods. You are essentially removing any foods that you could be sensitive to and that could be inflammatory or provoke a response from your immune system.

These foods include:

- Grains and starches
- Beans and legumes
- Dairy
- Eggs
- Nuts and seeds
- Nightshades (tomatoes, peppers, eggplant, etc.)
- Alcohol

While this list may seem extensive, don't worry! There are still plenty of foods you can enjoy during the elimination phase. In fact, you can eat every recipe in this book when you are in the AIP elimination phase. We want to make sure you can easily navigate this phase and never have to struggle to figure out what to eat for your next meal.

There is no set time frame for how long you should remain in the elimination phase. It really depends on the person. But we highly recommend staying in the elimination phase for a minimum of five weeks to allow your body sufficient time to heal.

The Reintroduction Phase

The autoimmune protocol isn't designed for you to stay in the elimination phase for the rest of your life. Once you start feeling well and your autoimmune symptoms have subsided, it's time for the reintroduction phase.

In general, most of our clients start the reintroduction phase between five and 12 weeks after beginning the elimination phase. Listen to your body and pay attention to its signals, such as cravings for certain types of foods or your intuition telling you that you are ready to reintroduce a food category. You will know when it is time.

The key to the reintroduction phase is doing it strategically, in stages. The goal is to slowly add specific foods in a specific order, and then allow sufficient time to see how your body reacts to those foods. It's really important during this phase to track everything you eat and all your symptoms so you can make an informed decision about what works for your body.

We have organized the reintroduction phase into five distinct stages. These stages are based on our own experience and what has worked best for us and our clients.

STAGE	FOODS TO REINTRODUCE
1	Non-AIP spices and ghee
2	Eggs and egg-based sauces
3	Seeds, nuts, and butter
4	Nightshades and dairy
5	Low-sugar alcohol and no-sugar-added sweeteners

The categories detailed in these stages correlate with the Foods to Eliminate, Then Reintroduce list on page 14 so you can see exactly which foods are in that category. Any food item that is considered inflammatory and is listed under Foods to Avoid on page 15 will not be on this list, because at the end of the day, we want you to continue on an anti-inflammatory diet. When you finish these five stages, you will have a customized list of foods you can eat that are tailored to your body's needs. How incredible is that?

When reintroducing foods, you need to take a measured approach. First, start with just *one* bite, slowly chew it, and then swallow. Wait 20 minutes and see if you experience any immediate reactions. If not, have a few more bites. Again, wait 20 minutes for any reactions or symptoms. If you still have no reactions, eat another few bites. This time, wait three hours for any reactions or symptoms to appear. If you still don't have any, eat a normal quantity of the food on just one day, and monitor for the next seven days.

During this seven-day period, don't reintroduce any other foods, and pay attention to body signals such as fatigue, digestive distress, headaches, poor sleep, joint pain, skin irritations, or mood changes, and check if any of your autoimmune symptoms have resurfaced. If, after seven days, you have no reactions or symptoms, you can reintroduce this food into your diet permanently. If at any time during this process you do experience a negative reaction or notice symptoms, mark this food as a No for reintroduction at this time.

If you have a really bad reaction to a food that doesn't subside, go back to the elimination phase before proceeding further. Remember, this is a journey, not a race. Take your time with the reintroduction phase.

Foods to Enjoy, Foods to Avoid

The table on page 11 is your reference guide throughout your autoimmune protocol. There are three sections in the table:

Foods to Eat Freely: These are foods that are AIP-friendly, meaning you can and should eat them in abundance. Once again, remember quality is key. Choose the highest quality and the most nutrient-dense foods available.

Foods to Eliminate, Then Reintroduce: These are foods you will remove from your diet in the elimination phase of the AIP. You will initially avoid these foods, but they can be slowly and carefully added back during the reintroduction phase.

Foods to Avoid: These are foods you should avoid now and going forward because they are inflammatory.

Foods to Eat Freely

PROTEINS

- Bacon, nitrate-free, no sugar added
- Beef
- Beef gelatin powder
- Bison
- Chicken
- Collagen peptides
- Crab
- Duck

- Elk
- Halibut
- Lamb
- Liver
- Lobster
- Mussels
- Oysters
- Pork
- Salmon

- Sardines
- Scallops
- Sea Bass
- Shrimp
- Squid
- Trout
- Tuna
- Turkey
- Tripe

FATS

- Avocado
- Avocado oil
- Bacon fat, nitrate-free, no sugar added
- Coconut butter, manna, and cream
- Coconut milk, full-fat unsweetened
- Coconut oil
- Extra-virgin olive oil
- Lard
- MCT oil
- Olives
- Palm shortening

VEGETABLES

- Artichokes
- Arugula
- Asparagus
- Bok choy
- Broccoli
- Brussels sprouts
- Butternut squash
- Cabbage
- Cauliflower
- Celery
- Chard
- Chives
- Cucumber
- Endive
- Fennel
- Garlic
- Kale
- Leeks
- Lettuce
- Mushrooms
- Okra
- Onions
- Plantains
- Potatoes
- Radicchio
- Radishes
- Rhubarb
- Shallots
- Spinach
- Sprouts
- Sweet potatoes
- Water chestnuts
- Zucchini

FRUITS

- Apples
- Bananas
- Blackberries
- Blueberries
- Cantaloupe
- Cherries
- Cranberries
- Dates
- Figs
- Grapefruits
- Grapes
- Kiwi
- Lemons
- Limes
- Mangos
- Oranges
- Peaches
- Pears
- Pineapples
- Plums
- Pomegranate seeds
- Raspberries
- Strawberries
- Watermelon

FERMENTED FOODS

- Kimchi
- Nondairy kefir
- Sauerkraut

BEVERAGES

- Bone broth
- Caffeinated black and green teas, unsweetened
- Herbal teas, such as chamomile, mint, rooibos, unsweetened
- Seltzer/sparkling water, unflavored
- Filtered water

HERBS AND SPICES

- Basil
- Bay leaf
- Chive
- Cilantro
- Cinnamon
- Clove
- Curry
- Dill
- Garlic
- Ginger
- Horseradish
- Lemongrass
- Oregano
- Parsley
- Peppermint
- Rose
- Rosemary
- Saffron
- Sage
- Salt, pink Himalayan and sea
- Spearmint
- Tarragon
- Thyme
- Turmeric
- Vanilla, powder and gluten-free extract

FLAVORINGS

- Capers
- Coconut aminos
- Fish sauce
- Vinegars: apple cider, balsamic, red wine, and white wine

NATURAL SWEETENERS

- Coconut sugar
- Molasses
- Pure maple syrup
- Raw honey

Foods to Eliminate, Then Reintroduce

NIGHTSHADES

- Eggplant
- Peppers of all kinds, including bell peppers, hot peppers, paprika, and cayenne
- Tomatillos
- Tomatoes

DAIRY

- Butter
- Buttermilk
- Cheese
- Cottage cheese
- Ghee
- Heavy cream
- Milk
- Sour cream
- Whey
- Yogurt, made from milk

EGGS AND EGG-BASED SAUCES

- Aioli
- Béarnaise
- Chicken eggs
- Duck eggs
- Mayonnaise

NUTS

- Almonds
- Brazil nuts
- Cashews
- Macadamia nuts
- Nut butters
- Nut milks
- Pecans
- Pine nuts
- Pistachios
- Walnuts

SEEDS

- Cacao
- Cocoa and chocolate
- Chia
- Coffee
- Flax
- Hemp
- Poppy
- Pumpkin
- Sesame
- Seed butters
- Seed milks
- Sunflower

NON-AIP SPICES

- Allspice
- Anise
- Caraway
- Cardamom
- Celery seed
- Coriander
- Cumin
- Dill seed
- Fennel seed
- Juniper
- Mustard seed
- Nutmeg
- Pepper, black and white

NO-SUGAR-ADDED SWEETENERS

- Erythritol, non-GMO
- Monk fruit extract, 100-percent pure
- Stevia, 100-percent pure

LOW-SUGAR ALCOHOL

- Clear liquors
- Dry wines

Foods to Avoid

GRAINS AND STARCHES

- Barley
- Buckwheat
- Corn
- Oats
- Quinoa
- Rice
- Rye
- Wheat

BEANS AND LEGUMES

- Beans
- Lentils
- Peanuts
- Peas

HIGH-SUGAR ALCOHOL

- Beer
- Dark liquors
- Hard ciders
- Sweet wines

REFINED OILS

- Canola
- Corn
- Grapeseed
- Margarine
- Soybean
- Vegetable

REFINED SUGARS

- Agave
- Brown sugar
- Evaporated cane juice
- High-fructose corn syrup
- Powdered sugar
- White sugar

ARTIFICIAL SWEETENERS AND DRINKS

- Energy drinks
- Equal
- Soda, including diet soda
- Splenda
- Sweet'N Low
- Truvía

SPOTLIGHT ON UNUSUAL INGREDIENTS

When creating the recipes in the book, we set out to make them as flavorful and delicious as possible. We also wanted to find innovative ways of taking classic dishes and making them AIP-friendly. We ended up using some ingredients you may not recognize. Below is a quick cheat sheet we created so you will know exactly what these ingredients are and where you can get them.

- **ARROWROOT STARCH:** This is extracted from the rhizomes of the arrowroot plant, and can be used as a substitute for cornstarch. It has no flavor of its own, making it the perfect thickener for sauces and soups. You can find it in the baking aisle at most grocery stores, or you can order it online.

- **BEEF GELATIN POWDER:** This is rendered from the bones of cows. It comes in powder form and is rich in collagen and amino acids; both are healing to your gut lining. When added to recipes, it acts as a thickener in sauces, yogurts, and custards. We like Great Lakes and Vital Proteins brands.

- **CASSAVA FLOUR:** This is the dried, peeled, and ground root of the cassava plant, and is the closest replacement for wheat flour that we have found. It's soft and powdery just like wheat flour, and for most recipes you can substitute it one-to-one. You can find cassava flour in the baking aisle at most grocery stores or you can order it online.

- **COCONUT AMINOS:** This liquid is made from the fermented sap of a coconut palm tree and combined with sea salt. Its salty and savory taste is similar to soy sauce, making it the perfect gluten-free and soy-free substitute. Our favorite brands are Coconut Secret, which is available at most grocery stores in the condiment aisle, or Thrive Market brand, which is available on their website.

- **COCONUT SUGAR:** This granulated sweetener is produced from coconut palm sap, and may also be called coconut palm sugar. It has the look and texture of brown sugar and can be substituted one-for-one for any type of granulated sweetener. You can find it in the baking aisle at most grocery stores, or you can order it online.

- **COLLAGEN PEPTIDES POWDER:** This powder is sourced from bovine hides or fish scales, and is full of amino acids that help support the health of your body's connective tissue, skin, hair, and nails. It has no taste, making it a great nutrient boost to add to smoothies and lattes.

- **FISH SAUCE:** This liquid condiment is made from fish that has been coated in salt and fermented. Even though the description doesn't sound too appealing, it actually provides incredible umami flavor in Asian dishes. Our favorite brand is Red Boat fish sauce. You can buy it in grocery stores, health food stores, Asian food markets, and online.

- **LARD:** This solid animal fat is mainly derived from pork. Lard is a great AIP substitute for butter. You can find it in jars in the cooking oil aisle of your local grocery store or online. Our favorite brands are Fatworks and Epic.

- **MCT OIL:** This liquid contains medium-chain triglycerides (MCTs) that are primarily extracted from coconut oil and are easily digestible. You can absorb MCTs in your bloodstream quickly, which results in fast energy. MCT oil is relatively flavorless, making it perfect to add to smoothies, salad dressings, and lattes for an extra dose of healthy fats.

- **SHIRATAKI NOODLES AND RICE:** These traditional Japanese noodles are made from the konjac yam, and are the perfect replacement for pasta and rice. Plus, they contain resistant starch (starch that is not digested in the small intestine), which fuels your good gut bacteria. They can be found in the refrigerated section of the grocery store, in Asian food markets, and online. Our favorite brand is Miracle Noodles.

- **TIGERNUT FLOUR:** This flour is made from ground tigernuts, which are small root vegetables that originated in Africa. They are a great source of vitamins E, C, and B_6, as well as resistant starch, which is a prebiotic that helps the good bacteria grow in the intestines. You can find the flour in health food stores or order it online.

- **VANILLA POWDER:** This powdered form of vanilla comes from ground vanilla beans and contains no alcohol or other added ingredients, which makes it perfect to add to smoothies, teas, and baked goods.

The Autoimmune Protocol Made Easy

This book is designed to set you up for success in following the autoimmune protocol. We have both been through our own healing journeys with autoimmune diseases and have taken everything we've learned and incorporated it into this book. In the following pages we are going to give you all the tools you need to heal your body from the inside so you can minimize or eliminate your autoimmune symptoms and truly live well.

We are going to start with preparation, which is essential for success. We will guide you through setting up your kitchen, shopping for the right foods, and prepping your meals. Once you are prepped and organized, we are providing you a sample meal plan to guide you through, especially if you are just starting out on the AIP.

Finally, we are sharing more than 100 AIP elimination phase recipes that are both simple to make and incredibly delicious, so that you always know what to eat and never feel stuck while doing AIP. The recipes were developed to be easy. Many require no cooking, are ready in 30 minutes or less, can be made in one pot or pan, or contain five ingredients or fewer (excluding salt, water, and oil)—or some mixture of all four. These easy labels will appear on the recipes for quick identification.

 NO COOK   ONE POT

 5 INGREDIENTS OR FEWER   30 MINUTES OR LESS

By the end of this book, you will feel confident, prepared, and motivated to start. This method completely changed our lives and transformed our health for the better, and we know it can do the same for you!

The AIP-Friendly Kitchen

Before you jump into the autoimmune protocol, we recommend getting your kitchen organized and optimized for this new way of life. Having an AIP-friendly kitchen really comes down to following just a few simple steps. You want to stock your kitchen with ingredients that are both versatile and used frequently in the recipes in this book. And you also want to ensure you have the kitchen equipment and tools on hand to prepare these recipes.

Pantry, Refrigerator, and Freezer Staples

If you want to fill your kitchen with nourishing foods, you first need to make room for them. This means a proper purge is in order. So grab a big bag and throw away or donate anything in your refrigerator, freezer, pantry, or kitchen cabinets that is on the Foods to Avoid List on page 15. Make sure to read the labels on any packaged foods to look for non-AIP ingredients. If you see an ingredient that you can't pronounce, that's a warning sign that it's not a real food! If you can't get rid of all of these items because your family or roommates want them, simply designate specific spaces in your refrigerator and pantry for storing these foods. This way, you can easily avoid these areas.

For some people, purging can be very liberating and motivating. Others find it to be extremely hard, as they feel like they are throwing away money and have doubts about what they are actually going to eat. Be strong and push through these emotions, knowing this step is crucial in setting yourself up for success. And don't worry—you will be replacing all these inflammatory items with nutrient-dense foods designed to heal your body!

On page 20 is a list of AIP staples that we use regularly and throughout the recipes in this book. Stocking your kitchen with these staples will ensure you have the basics to whip up an AIP-friendly meal any time.

- Coconut aminos
- Coconut milk, full-fat unsweetened
- Coconut oil

- Extra-virgin olive oil
- Apple cider vinegar
- Balsamic vinegar (no sugar added)

- Salt, pink Himalayan or sea

- Pastured chicken thighs
- Wild-caught salmon fillets (or any other fatty fish)

- Cauliflower (to make into rice or cauli-mash)
- Salad greens (spinach, kale, arugula)

- Vegetables (cucumber, broccoli, zucchini)
- Peeled whole garlic cloves (no added ingredients)

- Avocados

- Fresh herbs (basil, mint, rosemary, thyme)

- Lemons
- Limes
- Onions

Essential Equipment

AIP cooking doesn't require fancy equipment, but you do need a few basics to make the easy recipes in this book. You probably own most of these items already.

- Baking sheets
- Blender
- Cutting board
- Garlic press
- Grater
- Large stockpot with a lid
- Loaf pan

- Meat thermometer
- Mesh strainer
- Mixing bowls
- Muffin tin (12-cup)
- Parchment paper
- Saucepan with a lid
- Sharp knife

- Skillets (1 small, 1 large)
- Steamer basket
- Storage containers (airtight, various sizes)
- Utensils (peeler, spatula, strainer)

- Food processor
- Spiralizer
- Cheesecloth/ nut milk bag
- Slow cooker
- Handheld electric mixer
- Waffle iron

AIP-Friendly Cooking

Now that your kitchen is well-stocked, it's time to get cooking! Trust us, you don't have to be a professionally trained chef to master AIP-friendly cooking. During the elimination and reintroduction phases, you will be preparing most of your meals at home so you can control every ingredient and manage the quality of what you are eating. Below are our go-to tips for shopping and meal prep that will make cooking a breeze.

Shopping Made Simple

To eat quality, nutrient-dense foods, you first need to buy them. With that in mind, let's break down your shopping options.

GROCERY STORES

Most grocery stores offer quality organic foods. We recommend shopping the perimeter of the store and choosing organic items whenever possible.

Cost-Saving Tips:

- **BUY PRIVATE-LABEL.** Most supermarkets offer their own private-label organic foods. Because there is no middleman, the prices are cheaper. Just make sure they have the certified-organic seal.

- **TAKE ADVANTAGE OF SALES.** Shop store ads and look for the yellow sale tags, which often indicate a product is on sale.

- **BUY IN BULK.** When it comes to nuts, seeds, and even meat, buy them in bulk at a cheaper cost per pound. Portion out what you will use within a week and freeze the rest in airtight containers. Yes—even the nuts and seeds should go in the freezer. They will last for up to a year.

You can't beat the taste and nutrient profile of food that comes straight from a nearby farm. The shorter transport time ensures you are getting the food at its peak freshness. Make sure you seek out farmers who use organic farming techniques.

Cost-Saving Tips:

- **COMPARISON SHOP.** Do a walk of the entire market before you make any purchases, and compare the prices and quality among the vendors.

- **BUY SEASONAL PRODUCE.** Fruits and vegetables that are in season are generally the most affordable. Head to SeasonalFoodGuide.org to see what is in season in your area.

- **SHOP NEAR CLOSING TIME.** Some vendors will discount their prices right before closing time so they can sell off their produce rather than reload it on the truck.

ONLINE

Shopping online is a great option if you can't find quality foods at your local grocery store or farmers' market. It's also a good option if you're busy and don't have the time, you're sick and lack the energy to go to the store, or you simply like the convenience of having food delivered directly to your front door.

Cost-Saving Tips:

- **SHOP DISCOUNT WEBSITES.** There are many websites that offer quality products at affordable prices. Some of our favorites include Amazon, Thrive Market, Butcher Box, Sizzlefish, Vitacost, and Now Foods.

- **SIGN UP FOR OFFERS.** When prompted, provide your e-mail address so you get notified when there are sales or promo codes.

Meal Prep and Batch Cooking Basics

Meal prepping is a critical step to success, and will save time and energy on those days when you are super busy or just don't have the energy to cook. A big part of making things easy is making them in advance.

For the most part, you will need to carve out an hour or so on the weekend to get all your meal prepping done for the week. This includes washing and chopping your produce, roasting your proteins and vegetables all at once in a large batch, and making any soups, sauces, and dressings you'll want to use during the week. That way all you have to do is reheat and assemble meals throughout the week! Here are some tips for making your meal prep quick and easy.

- **WASH AND CHOP YOUR FRUITS AND VEGETABLES AS SOON AS YOU GET HOME FROM THE GROCERY STORE.** This will only take 15 or 20 minutes and will save so much time when you're cooking throughout the week.

- **HAVE PLENTY OF AIRTIGHT CONTAINERS ON HAND.** Clear glass storage containers are ideal, as they allow you to see exactly what's inside.

- **USE SIMILAR INGREDIENTS ACROSS MEALS, OR DOUBLE AND FREEZE.** When you're planning your meals for the week, look for ways to use the same ingredients in several recipes, or simply have the same meal more than once by cooking double or triple batches and refrigerating or freezing the leftovers. This way, you have fewer ingredients to buy and you can prep even more efficiently.

- **MAXIMIZE YOUR TIME BY BULK COOKING.** Cooking in bulk (also called batch cooking) is the most efficient way to use your time in the kitchen. Roast your proteins and vegetables in a large batch at the same time and store in the refrigerator to use another day.

- **PREP YOUR STAPLES.** Make any soups, sauces, recipe staples, and dressings to use during the week and across recipes.

Sample Meal Plan and Shopping List

The first trick to meal planning is to not overcomplicate it. For the first few weeks, keep your meals simple. Make a smoothie for breakfast, a soup for lunch, and a roasted protein with veggies for dinner. The simpler your meals are, the easier and faster it will be to prep them. This will also give you good practice and build your confidence. Once you master the basics, you can add recipes that take a little more time.

Use this sample meal plan to get started, or as a blueprint to make your own weekly meal plan. This meal plan can also be repeated or tweaked as you continue on your journey.

	BREAKFAST	LUNCH	DINNER
MONDAY	Berry and Kale Smoothie (page 73)	Tuscan Kale Soup (page 95)	Crispy-Skin Chicken Thighs with Coleslaw (page 134)
TUESDAY	Berry and Kale Smoothie (page 73)	Egg Roll in a Bowl (page 142)	Oven-Roasted Lemon Salmon and Asparagus (page 111)
WEDNESDAY	Berry and Kale Smoothie (page 73)	LEFTOVER Tuscan Kale Soup	LEFTOVER Crispy-Skin Chicken Thighs with Coleslaw
THURSDAY	Berry and Kale Smoothie (page 73)	LEFTOVER Egg Roll in a Bowl	LEFTOVER Oven-Roasted Lemon Salmon and Asparagus
FRIDAY	Berry and Kale Smoothie (page 73)	LEFTOVER Tuscan Kale Soup	LEFTOVER Crispy-Skin Chicken Thighs with Coleslaw
SATURDAY	Berry and Kale Smoothie (page 73)	LEFTOVER Egg Roll in a Bowl	Greek Steak Salad (page 104)
SUNDAY	Berry and Kale Smoothie (page 73)	LEFTOVER Tuscan Kale Soup	LEFTOVER Crispy-Skin Chicken Thighs with Coleslaw

Shopping List

PANTRY ITEMS

- Apple cider vinegar
- Avocado oil
- Coconut aminos
- Coconut sugar
- Collagen peptides powder
- Dried oregano
- Extra-virgin olive oil
- Salt, pink Himalayan or sea
- Raw honey
- White wine vinegar

ORGANIC PRODUCE

Fruits

- 1 avocado
- 4 bananas
- 3½ cups blackberries
- 3½ cups blueberries
- 1 lemon

Vegetables

- ½ pound asparagus
- 2 (14-ounce) bags coleslaw mix
- 3 carrots
- 3 stalks celery
- 8 cups lacinato kale
- 2 yellow onions
- 2 cups mixed greens
- 1 cucumber
- 1 red onion

Fresh herbs and spices

- 8 garlic cloves
- 2-inch piece fresh ginger

QUALITY PROTEINS

- 8 skin-on, bone-in chicken thighs
- 2 (6-ounce) salmon fillets
- 1½ pounds pork sausage (or can substitute ground pork)
- 1½ pounds ground pork
- 1 6-ounce skirt steak

LIQUIDS

- 6 cups chicken bone broth (store-bought or homemade, page 190)
- 3½ cups full-fat unsweetened coconut milk (store-bought or homemade, page 174)

The AIP-Friendly Life

Food plays an integral role in autoimmunity and healing, but there are also lifestyle factors you need to address to improve your health and minimize your symptoms. Here are some simple ways you can start to feel better on your AIP journey.

Sleep

Sufficient sleep is a ***must*** with the autoimmune protocol, as it is necessary for your physical and mental health. Aim for seven to nine hours each night. Here are some easy tips for improving your sleep.

- Create a bedtime ritual and follow it every night, with the goal of going to sleep at the same time every night.
- Put down your phone and turn off the TV at least two hours before your bedtime to avoid blue light exposure that can disrupt your sleep cycle.
- Improve your sleep environment by making sure your bedroom is quiet, dark, and cool.

Stress Management

Chronic and consistent stress can lead to health problems such as internal inflammation, hormone imbalance, and even a weakened immune system. Managing your stress is very important when it comes to your gut health. A few stress-relieving techniques you can employ at any time include sitting quietly and taking several slow, deep breaths; meditating; getting a massage or taking a bath; or taking up a relaxing hobby, such as painting, knitting, or gardening.

Movement

With AIP, we don't want you exercising too much and putting undue stress on your body. Over exercising or constantly pushing your body too hard, too long, or too often can do more harm than good. So, we just want you to focus on moving regularly, such as going for a walk outside, practicing yoga or Pilates, playing with your kids or pets, or stretching. It's important to really listen to your body. If you are feeling worn out or fatigued, slow down and rest.

Hydration

Here's the bottom line: You need to drink lots of water! At least ½ ounce for each pound that you weigh each day as a minimum. Always start your day with a large glass of water. If you are exercising and sweating, add even more water to your routine (at least another 24 ounces). To keep your electrolytes in balance, sprinkle your water with some pink Himalayan salt—it's a great source of electrolytes and, when combined with water, results in faster hydration. If you get bored with plain water, try some sparkling water. Or check out our recipes for Fruit and Herb Infused Water on page 32.

Exposure to Sunlight

For years now, we have been told to hide from the sun and slather on high-SPF sunscreen. But unfortunately, as a result of this advice, more and more people are becoming vitamin D-deficient. Vitamin D is essential for optimal health and plays a big role in immune system function. The best and most natural way to get vitamin D is to expose your skin to sunlight for 20 minutes each day before applying sunscreen. For people who don't live near the equator, year-round sun exposure is not possible. In this case, vitamin D supplementation is probably necessary. We recommend getting your vitamin D levels tested and working with a doctor to determine the best supplement dosage for you.

Eliminate Environmental Toxins

Toxins are not only in our foods, they're also in our household products, personal care items, and air and water supply. Taking in these toxins activates our immune system. To truly heal our immune system function, we need to eliminate as many as possible. Below are some of the best ways to do this.

Swap out your cleaning supplies. Choose natural cleaning products that use essential oils, vinegar, and other plant-based ingredients instead. Some of our favorite widely sold brands include The Honest Company, Seventh Generation, Branch Basics, and Mrs. Meyers Clean Day.

Upgrade your makeup and skin care products. Your skin is your body's largest organ and plays a crucial role in regulating your health. Every product that comes into contact with your skin has the potential to make its way into your bloodstream. Sadly, most skin care, hair care, and makeup companies use harmful ingredients in their products that can disrupt your endocrine system and impair immune function. Here are our favorite places to shop clean beauty brands: Credo Beauty (CredoBeauty.com), the Detox Market (TheDetoxMarket.com), Whole Foods (WholeFoodsMarket.com), and Honest Beauty (HonestBeauty.com).

Filter your water. Unfortunately, most standard tap water can be contaminated with toxins such as lead, arsenic, and radium. Use water filters to protect yourself from potentially harmful contaminants, such as a water filter pitcher or a faucet-attachment filter.

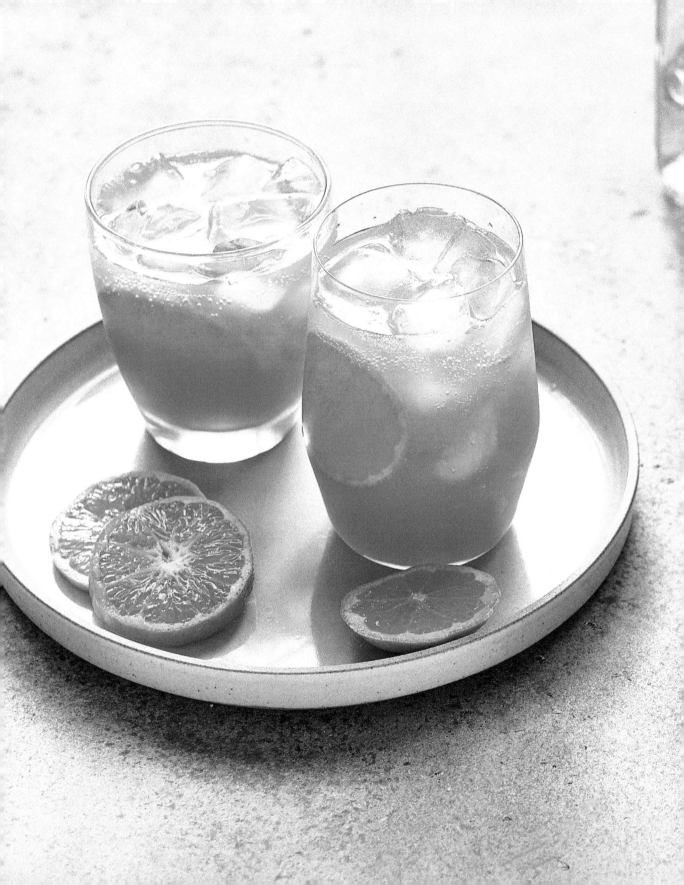

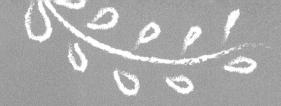

CHAPTER 2

DRINKS

Cranberry Orange Spritzer *page 34*

Fruit and Herb Infused Water

Hydration is a huge part of the autoimmune protocol. Some people find drinking plain water extremely boring, so we have come up with some fun flavor combinations you can use to make it more interesting.

FOR THE BASE

6 cups cold filtered water

STRAWBERRY BASIL

1 cup strawberries, trimmed and halved

¼ cup fresh basil leaves

CILANTRO LIME

2 limes, thinly sliced into circles

¼ cup fresh cilantro leaves

CUCUMBER MINT

½ cucumber, thinly sliced into circles

¼ cup fresh mint leaves

1. Combine the fruit and herb combination of your choice in a pitcher. Then pour in the water. Transfer to the refrigerator for 30 minutes so the flavors can infuse.

2. Serve over ice, if desired.

3. This water will stay fresh for 1 to 2 days in the refrigerator.

Make It Easier: You can also make flavored ice cubes to just drop into a glass or pitcher of plain water. Chop your herbs and thinly slice your fruit so that they can fit into the ice cube tray compartments. Fill the tray halfway with filtered water. Add the fruit and herbs, and use your fingers or a spoon to push them under the water. Put the half-filled ice cube tray in the freezer for about 1 hour. Add enough water to top up the cubes and freeze for 4 more hours, or until solid.

Per Serving: Calories: 0g; Total Fat: 0g; Total Carbs: 0g; Fiber: 0g; Net Carbs: 0g; Protein: 1g

Watermelon Cooler

Watermelon is one of the most hydrating foods you can eat, coming in at ½ cup of water for each 1 cup serving. Plus, it contains vitamin C, vitamin A, magnesium, and fiber. This drink is a delicious way to cool off and hydrate on a hot summer day.

1 cup watermelon, cubed, seeds removed

1 cup ice cubes

Juice of 1 lime

1 teaspoon coconut sugar (optional)

1. Put the watermelon, ice, lime juice, and coconut sugar (if using) in a blender and process until smooth.

2. Pour into a glass and serve. This drink is best enjoyed right away.

Swap or Substitute: Feel free to swap out the watermelon for an equal amount of honeydew or cantaloupe. If you prefer a smoother texture, you can use a mesh strainer to strain the blended drink into your glass.

Per Serving: Calories: 57; Total Fat: 0g; Total Carbs: 15g; Fiber: 1g; Net Carbs: 14g; Protein: 1g

Cranberry Orange Spritzer

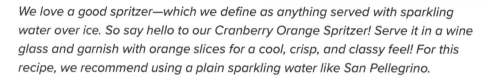

SERVES 1 / PREP TIME: 5 MINUTES

We love a good spritzer—which we define as anything served with sparkling water over ice. So say hello to our Cranberry Orange Spritzer! Serve it in a wine glass and garnish with orange slices for a cool, crisp, and classy feel! For this recipe, we recommend using a plain sparkling water like San Pellegrino.

2 cups sparkling water

¼ cup 100-percent pure cranberry juice

¼ cup 100-percent pure orange juice

Ice cubes

1. Pour the sparking water, cranberry juice, and orange juice into a wineglass and stir to combine.

2. Add as much ice as you like and enjoy. This drink is best served right away.

Swap or Substitute: Feel free to mix and match different fruit juice combinations based on what you have in your refrigerator. Just make sure you buy juice with only one ingredient (the fruit itself) and no added sugar.

Per Serving: Calories: 56; Total Fat: 0g; Total Carbs: 14g; Fiber: 0g; Net Carbs: 14g; Protein: 1g

ACV Citrus Tonic

Apple cider vinegar has many detoxifying and beneficial properties, including improving digestion, fighting kidney and bladder problems, and aiding in weight loss. On its own, the taste can be very sour, which is why this recipe uses fresh citrus and herbs to balance it out. Our sparkling water of choice for this recipe is San Pellegrino.

2 cups sparkling water

1 tablespoon apple cider vinegar

Juice of 1 lemon

1 teaspoon grated fresh ginger

1 teaspoon raw honey (optional)

Ice cubes

1. Pour the sparking water, vinegar, lemon juice, ginger, and honey (if using) into a large glass and stir to combine.

2. Add as much ice as you like and enjoy. This drink is best served right away.

Swap or Substitute: Add some additional flavors to your drink by muddling in fresh berries, mint, or basil.

Per Serving: Calories: 15; Total Fat: 0g; Total Carbs: 4g; Fiber: 0g; Net Carbs: 4g; Protein: 0g

Ginger Tea

When you're not feeling well, there is nothing better than a piping hot cup of ginger tea. This healthy tea is made with fresh ginger and is great for digestion and healing. Make a big batch by doubling or tripling this recipe. You can drink it cold or heat it up—whichever you prefer.

2-inch piece fresh ginger, peeled and sliced

2 cups filtered water

Juice of ½ lemon

1 teaspoon raw honey

1. In a medium saucepan, combine the ginger and water over high heat and gently boil for 15 minutes.

2. Remove the tea from the heat, stir in the lemon juice and honey, and enjoy.

3. Store any leftover tea in an airtight container in the refrigerator for up to 7 days.

Ingredient Spotlight: You will find fresh ginger in the produce section of most grocery stores. Choose a piece that is firm and pass on any that look wrinkled or appear moldy. If you have leftover ginger, freeze it to use later.

Per Serving: Calories: 30; Total Fat: 0g; Total Carbs: 8g; Fiber: 0g; Net Carbs: 8g; Protein: 0g

Raspberry Iced Green Tea

SERVES 4 / PREP TIME: 5 MINUTES
COOK TIME: 10 MINUTES / CHILL TIME: 1 HOUR

This is one of our favorite drinks. The earthy green tea pairs amazingly well with the sweet and tart berries. Raspberries contain beneficial phytonutrients and antioxidants, plus they are very high in vitamin C, making them the perfect addition to this drink. Check the tea bag ingredient list to make sure it doesn't contain sugar, soy lecithin, gluten, or other additives—just tea!

8 cups filtered water, divided

4 green tea bags

3 cups raspberries

Ice cubes

1. Heat 4 cups of water in a medium saucepan over high heat until it comes to boil. Add the tea bags and steep for 5 minutes.

2. In a separate large saucepan, heat the remaining 4 cups of water and the raspberries over high heat until it comes to a boil. Reduce the heat to low and simmer for 3 to 5 minutes, stirring regularly to break down the berries.

3. Pour the raspberry mixture through a mesh strainer into a large pitcher, followed by the brewed green tea. Stir to combine and transfer to the refrigerator to chill for at least 1 hour.

4. Pour into glasses full of ice to serve.

5. Store any leftover tea in the refrigerator for 1 to 2 days.

Swap or Substitute: Feel free to use frozen raspberries instead of fresh ones. To mix up the flavors, you can substitute an equal amount of strawberries, peaches, or even mango.

Per Serving: Calories: 17; Total Fat: 1g; Total Carbs: 1g; Fiber: 0g; Net Carbs: 1g; Protein: 1g

Turmeric Mango Lassi

SERVES 1 / PREP TIME: 5 MINUTES

Turmeric and its main active ingredient, curcumin, have powerful anti-inflammatory effects on the body. This drink features turmeric in a vibrant and refreshing way. The subtle sweetness of the mango pairs perfectly with the tanginess of the coconut yogurt. It's a bright and refreshing drink on a warm summer day.

½ cup filtered water

½ cup cubed frozen mango

½ cup plain unsweetened coconut yogurt

1 teaspoon ground turmeric

1. Put the water, mango, coconut yogurt, and turmeric in a blender and process until smooth.

2. Pour into a glass and serve. This drink is best enjoyed right away.

Ingredient Spotlight: When buying coconut yogurt, make sure the only ingredients are coconut, water, and probiotic cultures. We like the brands Anita's and GT's CocoYo.

Per Serving: Calories: 134; Total Fat: 4g; Total Carbs: 20g; Fiber: 2g; Net Carbs: 18g; Protein: 5g

Frozen Piña Colada Slushy

This drink is our AIP-friendly version of a piña colada. It is tropical, coconutty, and just plain good. You can easily increase this recipe to serve a crowd.

½ cup coconut cream

½ cup 100-percent pure pineapple juice

½ cup frozen pineapple chunks

3 cups ice

Pineapple wedge for garnish (optional)

1. Put the coconut cream, pineapple juice and chunks, and ice in a blender and process until smooth.

2. Pour into a glass, garnish with a pineapple wedge (if using), and serve. This drink is best enjoyed right away.

Swap or Substitute: You can find coconut cream at your local grocery store; it usually comes in a can. Make sure the only ingredients are coconut and water. If you can't find coconut cream, skim off the solid white cream that rises to the top of a can of full-fat unsweetened coconut milk and use that instead.

Per Serving: Calories: 504; Total Fat: 42g; Total Carbs: 35g; Fiber: 4g; Net Carbs: 31g; Protein: 5g

Cleansing Green Juice

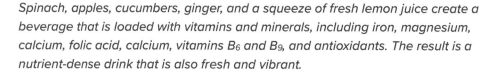

SERVES 1 / PREP TIME: 5 MINUTES / COOK TIME: 5 MINUTES

Spinach, apples, cucumbers, ginger, and a squeeze of fresh lemon juice create a beverage that is loaded with vitamins and minerals, including iron, magnesium, calcium, folic acid, calcium, vitamins B_6 and B_9, and antioxidants. The result is a nutrient-dense drink that is also fresh and vibrant.

1 cup cold filtered water

1 cup baby spinach

1 green apple, cored and quartered

½ cucumber, peeled and quartered

1-inch piece fresh ginger, peeled

Juice of 1 lemon

1. Put the water, spinach, apple, cucumber, ginger, and lemon in a blender and process until smooth.

2. Pour into a glass and serve. This drink is best enjoyed right away.

Swap or Substitute: If you prefer a smoother texture, you can use a mesh strainer to strain the blended drink into your glass.

Per Serving: Calories: 136; Total Fat: 1g; Total Carbs: 35g; Fiber: 6g; Net Carbs: 29g; Protein: 3g

Golden Milk

SERVES 1 / PREP TIME: 5 MINUTES / COOK TIME: 5 MINUTES

This healing Golden Milk is especially comforting on a cold winter's day. The turmeric, ginger, and cinnamon are a classic combination and provide a warming flavor. The coconut milk and coconut oil provide plenty of medium-chain fatty acids, which the body absorbs easily and uses for energy.

1½ cups full-fat unsweetened coconut milk (store-bought or homemade, page 174)

1 teaspoon ground turmeric

⅛ teaspoon ground ginger

⅛ teaspoon cinnamon

2 teaspoons coconut oil

1 teaspoon raw honey (optional)

1. In a medium saucepan, combine the coconut milk, turmeric, ginger, cinnamon, coconut oil, and honey (if using) over medium heat and whisk well. Remove from the heat when the liquid is hot but not boiling.

2. Pour into a large mug and serve.

3. Store any leftovers in an airtight container in the refrigerator for up to 7 days.

Make It Easier: You can also enjoy this drink cold. We like to double or triple the batch and keep it in the refrigerator for a quick anti-inflammatory drink.

Per Serving: Calories: 879; Total Fat: 81g; Total Carbs: 12g; Fiber: 1g; Net Carbs: 11g; Protein: 7g

Vanilla Date Milk

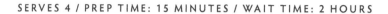

SERVES 4 / PREP TIME: 15 MINUTES / WAIT TIME: 2 HOURS

We are obsessed with this Vanilla Date Milk and use it all the time. We add it in place of coconut milk in our Pumpkin Spice Smoothie (page 69) and Cinnamon Apple Smoothie (page 72). We also pour it over our On-the-Go Granola (page 75) for a quick breakfast.

4 cups filtered water

2 cups unsweetened shredded coconut

4 dates, pitted

1 tablespoon pure vanilla powder

1. Heat the filtered water in a large saucepan over medium heat. When the water starts to simmer, remove it from the heat. Do not boil. Transfer the water to a large bowl and add the coconut and dates. Let sit for 1 to 2 hours.

2. Pour the mixture into a blender. Blend on the highest speed for about 1 minute, or until fully combined. Strain through a nut milk bag or a piece of cheesecloth (you can use a coffee filter or very thin dish towel in a pinch) and squeeze all the liquid from the strainer.

3. Pour the liquid back into the blender and add the vanilla powder. Process until smooth.

4. Pour into a glass and enjoy, or transfer to an air-tight container and store in the refrigerator for up to 5 days.

Ingredient Spotlight: During the elimination phase of the AIP, avoid using vanilla extract in raw-food recipes in which the alcohol will not cook off. Instead, choose pure vanilla powder, which you can find online or at most health food stores.

Creamy Carob "Coffee"

SERVES 1 / PREP TIME: 10 MINUTES / COOK TIME: 5 MINUTES

Coffee is one of the hardest things to eliminate on the AIP diet. Fortunately, there are some great alternatives that mimic the look and flavor of coffee. This drink features two ingredients that come very close—carob and chicory root. Carob is available in powder form and has a flavor similar to cocoa. Chicory root is part of the dandelion family and tastes like coffee. This recipe may seem a little complex, but it's actually very easy. You're just making a cup of chicory coffee, heating up the coconut milk, and mixing them in the blender.

1 cup filtered water

2 tablespoons ground chicory

1 cup full-fat unsweetened coconut milk (store-bought or homemade, page 174)

1 tablespoon carob powder

1 teaspoon cinnamon, plus more for garnish

1 teaspoon coconut sugar (optional)

Ingredient Spotlight:
You can find both carob powder and chicory root in many grocery stores, at your local health food store, or online. Make sure to check the ingredient list to be sure neither contains any sugar, soy lecithin, gluten, or other additives. There should be only one ingredient each.

1. Bring the water to a boil in a kettle or small saucepan over high heat. Add the chicory root to the bottom of a large mug or teapot and pour in the boiling water. Steep for 4 to 5 minutes.

2. Heat the coconut milk in a small saucepan over medium heat until the mixture comes to a light simmer. Remove from the heat and pour into a blender. Add the carob powder, cinnamon, and coconut sugar (if using). Using a mesh strainer, pour the chicory root mixture into the blender.

3. Blend for 10 to 30 seconds, or until fully combined. The liquid will be hot, so place a dish towel over the top of the blender before turning it on.

4. Pour the mixture into a large mug, garnish with more cinnamon, and serve. This drink is best enjoyed right away.

Per Serving: Calories: 464; Total Fat: 49g; Total Carbs: 11g; Fiber: 3g; Net Carbs: 8g; Protein: 6g

Bone Broth Latte

SERVES 1 / PREP TIME: 5 MINUTES / COOK TIME: 3 MINUTES

Bone broth is incredibly healing and restorative to the lining of your gut. We recommend drinking it daily, and one of the easiest ways to do that is with this latte. Make sure to heat your bone broth on the stovetop so it's nice and warm.

1 cup Chicken Bone Broth (store-bought or homemade, page 190)

1 tablespoon Garlic-Infused Oil (page 180)

1 teaspoon lemon juice

Pinch pink Himalayan salt or sea salt

1. Heat the bone broth in a small saucepan until it's hot. Do not boil.

2. Pour the broth in a blender and add the oil, lemon juice, and salt, then blend for 10 to 30 seconds, or until fully combined. The liquid will be hot, so place a dish towel over the top of the blender before turning it on.

3. Pour into a mug and enjoy warm. This drink is best served right away.

Swap or Substitute: You can use any type of bone broth in this recipe (beef, chicken, or a combo). If you don't have time to make a batch of homemade bone broth, you can use store-bought. Check the ingredients label to make sure all the ingredients are AIP-friendly. We like Bonafide Provisions or Kettle & Fire brands.

Per Serving: Calories: 135; Total Fat: 14g; Total Carbs: 1g; Fiber: 0g; Net Carbs: 1g; Protein: 2g

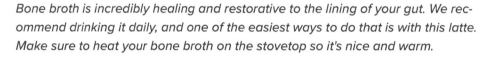
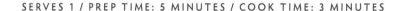

Cinnamon Coconut Matcha Latte

SERVES 1 / PREP TIME: 8 MINUTES / COOK TIME: 5 MINUTES

This drink will soon be your morning staple. It's packed with natural energy and healthy fats to keep you fueled. Matcha, a finely ground powder of special green tea leaves, is full of antioxidants, including EGCG (epigallocatechin gallate), which is believed to reduce inflammation and is rich in fiber, chlorophyll, and other nutrients.

1 cup full-fat unsweetened coconut milk (store-bought or homemade, page 174)

1 teaspoon matcha powder

2 tablespoons hot filtered water

1 tablespoon collagen peptides powder

1 teaspoon MCT oil

1 teaspoon cinnamon, plus more for garnish

1 teaspoon raw honey (optional)

1. Heat the coconut milk in a medium saucepan over medium heat until it comes to a light simmer.

2. Pour the matcha powder in a small bowl. Add the water. Using the back of a spoon or a bamboo whisk, stir the mixture into a paste. Once the coconut milk is simmering, remove the saucepan from the heat and stir in the matcha paste.

3. Transfer the mixture to a blender and add the collagen powder, MCT oil, cinnamon, and honey (if using). The liquid will be hot, so place a dish towel over the top of the blender before turning it on. Blend for 10 to 30 seconds, or until fully combined.

4. Pour into a large mug and sprinkle with cinnamon. This drink is best served right away.

Ingredient Spotlight: Be sure to use full-fat coconut milk with no additives. The only ingredients should be coconut and water. We like Native Forest Simple Coconut Milk, which comes in a can. Also, make sure to shake the can vigorously before opening to combine the coconut and water.

Per Serving: Calories: 525; Total Fat: 52g; Total Carbs: 8g; Fiber: 1g; Net Carbs: 7g; Protein: 14g

Earl Grey Latte

Earl Grey tea contains bergamot oil, a powerful polyphenol that is known for its natural healing properties and for promoting cellular regeneration. This latte is incredibly rich and creamy, and it will keep you satisfied and energized all morning. This recipe may seem a little busy, but it's really not. You're just making a cup of tea, heating up the coconut milk, and mixing them in the blender.

½ cup filtered water

1 Earl Grey tea bag

1 cup full-fat unsweetened coconut milk (store-bought or homemade, page 174)

1 teaspoon gluten-free vanilla extract

1 tablespoon collagen peptides powder

1 teaspoon MCT oil

1 teaspoon raw honey (optional)

1. Bring the water to a boil in a kettle or small saucepan over high heat. Pour the boiling water into a large mug or teapot. Add the tea bag and steep for 4 to 5 minutes.

2. Heat the coconut milk and vanilla in a small saucepan over medium heat until the mixture comes to a light simmer. Pour the mixture into a blender. Add the collagen powder, MCT oil, and honey (if using).

3. Discard the tea bag and pour the tea into the blender. Blend for 10 to 30 seconds or until fully combined. The liquids will be hot, so place a dish towel over the top of the blender before turning it on.

4. Pour the latte into a large mug and serve. This drink is best enjoyed right away.

Ingredient Spotlight: When choosing your Earl Grey tea bags, look for organic varieties and make sure the only ingredients are black tea and bergamot oil. Choose gluten-free vanilla extract, as grain alcohol is often used in vanilla extract. The alcohol will cook off when heated, so vanilla extract works in the elimination phase of AIP.

Per Serving: Calories: 531; Total Fat: 52g; Total Carbs: 7g; Fiber: 0g; Net Carbs: 7g; Protein: 14g

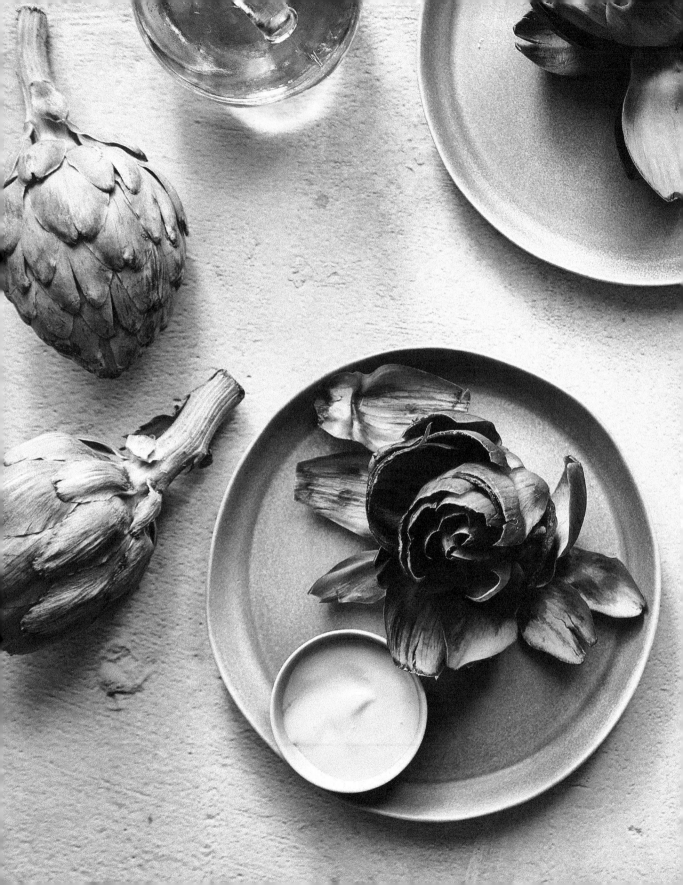

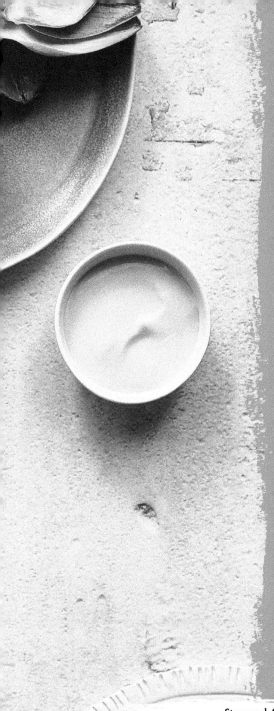

SMALL BITES AND SNACKS

**Steamed Artichokes with
Creamy Balsamic Dipping Sauce** *page 54*

Prosciutto-Wrapped Melon

SERVES 4 / PREP TIME: 10 MINUTES

This easy and classic appetizer is a little sweet, a little salty, and comes together quickly. Cantaloupe is loaded with beta-carotene, which converts to vitamin A and acts as a powerful antioxidant. It also contains vitamin C, folate, fiber, and potassium, which can aid in nerve and muscle health.

½ ripened cantaloupe

3 ounces (about 5 slices) prosciutto, thinly sliced

1 teaspoon raw honey

½ teaspoon fresh thyme leaves (optional)

1. Using a sharp knife, trim the rind from the melon and cut it into 2-by-2-inch pieces.

2. Tear the prosciutto into strips and wrap each strip around a piece of melon.

3. Arrange the wrapped melon on a plate and drizzle with the honey. Sprinkle the thyme on top, if using, and enjoy.

4. Store any leftovers in an airtight container in the refrigerator for up to 3 to 4 days.

Swap or Substitute: You can replace the cantaloupe with honeydew, dates, or pears.

Per Serving: Calories: 41; Total Fat: 2g; Total Carbs: 2g; Fiber: 0g; Net Carbs: 2g; Protein: 4g

Crispy Kale Chips

SERVES 4 / PREP TIME: 5 MINUTES / COOK TIME: 15 MINUTES

Crispy Kale Chips are the perfect snack when you need a salty, crunchy bite. The antioxidants in kale, including quercetin and kaempferol, have anti-inflammatory properties that make them a perfect vegetable for those suffering from auto-immune disease. Make a big batch and have these chips on hand to snack on throughout the week.

2 pounds curly kale

3 tablespoons avocado oil

½ teaspoon pink Himalayan salt or sea salt

1. Preheat the oven to 375°F. Line a large baking sheet with parchment paper.

2. Lay each kale leaf on a cutting board and cut out the thick center stem. Tear the larger leaves into smaller pieces.

3. In a large bowl, toss the kale with the avocado oil and salt. Spread out the kale in a single layer on the baking sheet and bake for 15 minutes, or until crisp. Allow the chips to cool before enjoying.

4. Store leftover chips in an airtight container at room temperature for up to 1 week.

Ingredient Spotlight: Make sure to use curly kale in this recipe. The leaves are much sturdier than lacinato kale and make for a crisper chip.

Per Serving: Calories: 209; Total Fat: 13g; Total Carbs: 20g; Fiber: 8g; Net Carbs: 12g; Protein: 10g

Baked Cinnamon Apple Chips

SERVES 4 / PREP TIME: 8 MINUTES
COOK TIME: 2 HOURS / COOLING TIME: 30 MINUTES

These apple chips will definitely satisfy your sweet tooth. They make a perfect quick snack and are also a great addition to a charcuterie board. We also love using them in our On-the-Go Granola (page 75). Baking these slowly at a low temperature ensures they crisp up perfectly every time. Just pop them in the oven, set a timer, and let your oven do all the work.

3 Honeycrisp apples

½ teaspoon cinnamon

1. Preheat the oven to 200°F. Line two large baking sheets with parchment paper.

2. Core the apples using an apple corer, then cut them into ⅛-inch-thick slices using a mandoline or a very sharp knife. Lay the slices on the baking sheets in a single layer, without overlapping. Sprinkle the cinnamon evenly over the slices.

3. Bake for 2 hours. Test the doneness by removing one slice and letting it sit out at room temperature for a few minutes. If it's crispy, remove the apple chips from the oven.

4. Cool for 30 minutes to allow the chips to crisp up fully.

5. Store leftovers in an airtight container at room temperature for up to 7 days.

Swap or Substitute: Feel free to swap the Honeycrisp apples in this recipe for your favorite variety—Red Delicious, Fuji, or Gala are great options.

Per Serving: Calories: 72; Total Fat: 0g; Total Carbs: 19g; Fiber: 3g; Net Carbs: 16g; Protein: 0g

Thyme Zucchini Chips

Crispy and lightly seasoned, zucchini chips make the perfect alternative to potato chips or crackers. And they're so easy to make. Just slice, season, and go do something else as they slowly bake in the oven. These chips taste great on their own, or you can serve them up with your favorite AIP-friendly dip.

4 zucchini, thinly sliced

2 tablespoons
avocado oil, divided

½ teaspoon pink
Himalayan salt or sea salt

½ teaspoon garlic powder

½ teaspoon dried
thyme or 2 teaspoons
chopped fresh thyme

1. Spread the zucchini slices on paper towels without overlapping. Place a large baking sheet on top of the paper towels to help press out any moisture. Let sit for 15 minutes.

2. Preheat the oven to 235°F. Line the same baking sheet with parchment paper. Brush 1 tablespoon avocado oil on the parchment.

3. Arrange the zucchini slices on the lined baking sheet in a single layer and brush the remaining 1 tablespoon of avocado oil on top of the slices. In a small bowl, mix together the salt, garlic powder, and thyme. Sprinkle on top of the zucchini slices.

4. Bake for 1½ to 2 hours, or until crisp and golden brown. Allow the chips to cool before enjoying.

5. Store leftovers in an airtight container at room temperature for up to 3 days.

Ingredient Spotlight: When choosing the zucchini, look for a wide diameter, as the chips will shrink considerably during baking.

Per Serving: Calories: 97; Total Fat: 7g; Total Carbs: 6g; Fiber: 2g; Net Carbs: 4g; Protein: 2g

Steamed Artichokes with Creamy Balsamic Dipping Sauce

SERVES 2 / PREP TIME: 5 MINUTES / COOK TIME: 25 MINUTES

The cynarin in artichokes aids in digestion and can significantly improve IBS symptoms—which make this wonderful vegetable perfect for anyone suffering from autoimmune disease. Steaming is the best way to prepare artichokes, and our foolproof method results in perfectly cooked artichokes every time.

2 artichokes

½ lemon

1½ teaspoons pink Himalayan salt or sea salt

¼ cup plain unsweetened coconut yogurt

2 tablespoons balsamic vinegar

1 tablespoon extra-virgin olive oil

1 tablespoon lemon juice

2 teaspoons raw honey

Pinch pink Himalayan salt or sea salt

1. Prepare the artichokes as described in the Ingredient Spotlight (page 55) and rub the cut surfaces with the lemon to prevent discoloration.

2. Set a steamer basket in a large pot and add enough filtered water to fill the pot just below the basket. Squeeze the juice from the lemon half into the pot and add the salt. Bring to a boil.

3. Place the artichokes in the steamer basket stem-side up. Cover the pot and steam for 25 minutes, or until the artichoke hearts are tender when pierced with a tip of a paring knife and the inner leaves pull out easily.

4. While the artichokes are steaming, make the sauce by whisking together the yogurt, vinegar, oil, lemon juice, honey, and salt in a small bowl.

5. Serve the steamed artichokes with the dipping sauce on the side.

6. Store any leftovers in an airtight container in the refrigerator for up to 5 days.

Ingredient Spotlight: Look for plump artichokes with tight leaves and firm stems. The heavier the artichoke is for its size, the better it will taste. Avoid artichokes with dried and split leaves. Prepare them by snapping off the tough outer leaves. Use a serrated knife to cut off the top third, then use kitchen shears to snip off the remaining spiky leaf tips. Trim the stems so the artichokes stand upright.

Per Serving: Calories: 194; Total Fat: 8g; Total Carbs: 28g; Fiber: 9g; Net Carbs: 19g; Protein: 6g

Bacon-Wrapped Water Chestnuts

SERVES 4 / PREP TIME: 5 MINUTES / COOK TIME: 45 MINUTES

These bite-size snacks are crunchy and flavorful, making them a crowd-pleasing appetizer to serve at a party. Water chestnuts contain a surprisingly high amount of fiber—3 grams per serving—which can help promote a healthy gut. If you don't have time to make the AIP Barbecue Sauce (page 186), you can buy an AIP-friendly brand (we recommend KC Natural Mastodon) or simply leave it out. They will still taste great!

1 pound bacon,
slices cut in half

2 (8-ounce) cans whole water chestnuts, drained

1 cup AIP Barbecue Sauce (page 186) or store-bought barbecue sauce

1. Preheat the oven to 375°F. Line a large baking sheet with aluminum foil.

2. Wrap each water chestnut with a half slice of bacon and secure it with a toothpick. Place the speared water chestnuts on the baking sheet.

3. Bake for 15 minutes. Drain the bacon grease from the baking sheet and brush each water chestnut with the barbecue sauce. Bake for another 30 minutes, or until the bacon is crispy and browned. Serve warm.

4. Store any leftovers in an airtight container in the refrigerator for up to 3 to 4 days.

Ingredient Spotlight: Make sure to check the ingredients on the bacon package to ensure any added seasoning is AIP-friendly.

Per Serving: Calories: 618; Total Fat: 30g; Total Carbs: 55g; Fiber: 4g; Net Carbs: 51g; Protein: 31g

Shrimp Ceviche

SERVES 4 / PREP TIME: 10 MINUTES
COOK TIME: 1 MINUTE / CHILL TIME: 1 HOUR

Light and refreshing, this shrimp ceviche makes for great appetizer or a light lunch. Our version features vibrant citrus juice and creamy avocado for the perfect balance of flavors. The shrimp actually "cooks" by just resting in the citrus juice, which gives you time to relax instead of working in the kitchen. This dish can be made up to 8 hours in advance. It pairs perfectly with our AIP Garlic Herb Flatbread (page 62).

1 pound small shrimp, peeled and deveined

¾ cup lemon juice

¾ cup lime juice

½ cup finely diced red onion

1 cucumber, diced

1 avocado, pitted, peeled, and diced

¼ cup chopped fresh cilantro

1. Bring a large pot of filtered water to a boil and cook the shrimp for 30 to 45 seconds. Drain the shrimp into a colander, and run cold water over them to stop them from cooking any further.

2. Transfer the shrimp to a large glass bowl and add the lemon and lime juice. Gently toss to fully coat the shrimp, cover the bowl, and refrigerate for 1 hour.

3. Mix in the onion, cucumber, avocado, and cilantro, stirring gently to combine.

4. Serve chilled.

5. Store any leftovers in an airtight container in the refrigerator for up to 3 to 4 days.

Ingredient Spotlight: For the best flavor, buy fresh shrimp from the seafood counter. We prefer to use small, bite-size shrimp to make the ceviche easier to eat, but you can also use larger shrimp and cut them into smaller pieces.

Per Serving: Calories: 205; Total Fat: 9g; Total Carbs: 16g; Fiber: 5g; Net Carbs: 11g; Protein: 18g

Grilled Oysters with Lemon

SERVES 4 / PREP TIME: 5 MINUTES / COOK TIME: 10 MINUTES

This simple and elegant oyster dish makes the perfect appetizer or snack. Oysters are rich in zinc, omega-3 fatty acids, potassium, magnesium, selenium, iron, and vitamins A, E, C, and B₁₂, which make them perfect for an anti-inflammatory diet. Don't be intimidated to cook these—the grilling process will pop the shells open for you. If you don't have access to an outdoor grill, add them to a roasting pan filled with ⅓ inch water and bake at 475°F for 7 to 10 minutes.

24 fresh raw oysters
in their shells

Juice of ½ lemon

Pinch pink Himalayan
salt or sea salt

1. Preheat the grill to high.

2. Place the oysters on the grill with the flatter side up. Cook for 5 to 10 minutes, or until they pop open.

3. Carefully remove the top shell, leaving the oyster in the bottom shell.

4. Squeeze lemon juice evenly over the oysters. Sprinkle with salt and enjoy immediately.

Ingredient Spotlight: Discard any oysters that have opened before cooking and any that are unopened after cooking. You will usually get several oysters that are not safe to eat, so always buy more than you think you'll need. Use a grill mitt and tongs to handle the hot shells. When prying open the oysters, try to keep the oyster liquor inside the shell—it has a lovely flavor.

Per Serving: Calories: 51; Total Fat: 1g; Total Carbs: 4g; Fiber: 0g; Net Carbs: 4g; Protein: 4g

Citrus-Marinated Smoked Salmon

SERVES 4 / PREP TIME: 5 MINUTES / CHILL TIME: 25 MINUTES

Smoked salmon is the perfect no-cook option when you need a quick snack or a simple appetizer. Salmon contains vitamin D, and getting sunlight regularly or eating foods rich in vitamin D should be a part of your daily routine, especially when you have an autoimmune condition. This dish pairs well with our AIP Garlic Herb Flatbread (page 62).

Zest and juice of 1 lemon

2 tablespoons extra-virgin olive oil

2 tablespoons coconut aminos

8 ounces sliced smoked salmon

2 radishes, thinly sliced

1 scallion, chopped (optional)

1. In a baking dish, whisk together the lemon zest, lemon juice, olive oil, and coconut aminos.

2. Place the salmon in the dish. Cover and marinate in the refrigerator for 25 minutes, flipping halfway through.

3. Arrange the salmon, radishes, and scallions (if using) to serve.

4. Store any leftovers in an airtight container in the refrigerator for up to 3 to 4 days.

Ingredient Spotlight: Avoid smoked salmon that has dark brown spots around the edges. This is a sign that it is a lower-quality product and may have added sugars. Whenever possible, choose wild-caught smoked salmon with no added ingredients except salt.

Per Serving: Calories: 108; Total Fat: 7g; Total Carbs: 1g; Fiber: 0g; Net Carbs: 1g; Protein: 9g

Collagen Protein Bars

MAKES 8 BARS / PREP TIME: 10 MINUTES / CHILL TIME: 20 MINUTES

These no-cook snack bars are healthy, easy, and delicious. Collagen bars are a perfect way to get collagen into your diet. Collagen is a structural protein that is known to decrease gut permeability; improve the appearance of your skin, nails, and hair; and decrease inflammation in your joints.

1 cup dried dates, pitted

1 cup dried cranberries

½ cup collagen peptides powder

¼ teaspoon pink Himalayan salt or sea salt

2 tablespoons coconut oil

1. Line an 8-by-8-inch baking pan with parchment paper, leaving an overhang for easy lifting.

2. Combine the dates and cranberries in a blender or food processor and pulse until chopped completely. Add the collagen powder, salt, and coconut oil and pulse until fully combined.

3. Transfer the mixture to the lined baking pan and press it down into an even layer. Place the pan in the freezer for 20 minutes, or until firm.

4. Remove from the baking pan by lifting the parchment paper. Cut into 8 bars.

5. Store in an airtight container at room temperature for up to 7 days.

Swap or Substitute: Be careful with the dried cranberries, which often are sold with added sugar. You can experiment with different flavors by swapping them for dried cherries or dried blueberries.

Per Serving (1 bar): Calories: 164; Total Fat: 4g; Total Carbs: 26g; Fiber: 2g; Net Carbs: 24g; Protein: 10g

Blueberry Granola Bars

MAKES 8 BARS / PREP TIME: 5 MINUTES
COOK TIME: 10 MINUTES / CHILL TIME: 1 TO 2 HOURS

You'll love having these AIP-friendly granola bars on hand when you want a quick snack. Most store-bought granola bars are made with grains and nuts, but our anti-inflammatory version uses coconut chips and dried fruit. This recipe requires the bars to set in the refrigerator for 1 to 2 hours, but they are definitely worth the wait because the result is pure deliciousness.

2 cups coconut chips

½ cup dried blueberries

¼ cup chopped dried apricots

4 tablespoons coconut oil, divided

1 tablespoon raw honey

1 tablespoon cinnamon

½ teaspoon pink Himalayan salt or sea salt

1¼ cups coconut butter, melted

1 tablespoon collagen peptides powder

1. Preheat the oven to 350°F. Line a baking sheet and an 8-by-8-inch baking pan with parchment paper.

2. Mix together the coconut chips, blueberries, apricots, 2 tablespoons of coconut oil, honey, cinnamon, and salt on the baking sheet. Spread the mixture in an even layer and bake for 10 minutes.

3. Remove the granola from the oven, transfer it to the baking pan, and mix in the remaining 2 tablespoons coconut oil, coconut butter, and collagen powder. Press the mixture firmly into the pan in an even layer.

4. Refrigerate the pan for 1 to 2 hours, or until hardened. Remove from the refrigerator and let soften for 15 minutes before cutting into bars.

5. Store in an airtight container at room temperature for up to 7 days.

Ingredient Spotlight: Coconut butter may also be called coconut manna, and is not the same as coconut oil. It comes in a jar and can be found online or near the coconut oil in the grocery store or health food store. You can also make you own with dried shredded coconut. Put 4 cups in a food processor or blender and process continuously for 5 to 10 minutes, until a creamy butter forms.

Per Serving (1 bar): Calories: 447; Total Fat: 37g; Total Carbs: 26g; Fiber: 9g; Net Carbs: 17g; Protein: 5g

AIP Garlic Herb Flatbread

MAKES 4 FLATBREADS / PREP TIME: 10 MINUTES / COOK TIME: 30 MINUTES

Yes, you read correctly! This is our version of flatbread, made AIP-friendly. It's delicious on its own, and also tastes amazing topped with arugula, pesto, prosciutto, olive oil, or avocado. Or serve it as an accompaniment to Citrus-Marinated Smoked Salmon (page 59), Shrimp Ceviche (page 57), Smoked Salmon with Avocado (page 82), or any dish where you miss having bread on the side.

1½ cups full-fat unsweetened coconut milk (store-bought or homemade, page 174)

¾ cup cassava flour

¾ cup arrowroot starch

¼ teaspoon pink Himalayan salt or sea salt

½ teaspoon dried rosemary or 2 teaspoons chopped fresh rosemary

1 teaspoon dried garlic flakes, divided

1. In a medium bowl, mix together the coconut milk, cassava flour, arrowroot flour, and salt.

2. Heat a medium skillet over medium heat. Pour in one-quarter of the batter and tilt the pan from side to side to distribute it evenly. Sprinkle with the rosemary and garlic flakes.

3. Cook for 3 to 4 minutes, then use a wide spatula to flip the bread and cook for another 3 to 4 minutes. Increase the heat if it takes longer than 4 minutes to start browning, and reduce it if the bread starts to blacken.

4. Repeat for the remaining three flatbreads. Enjoy warm.

5. Store leftovers in an airtight container at room temperature for up to 3 to 4 days or in the refrigerator for up to 5 days. You can also store the flatbread in the freezer for up to 3 months.

Ingredient Spotlight: Cassava flour comes from the cassava root and is the closest replacement for wheat flour that we've found. Arrowroot starch is extracted from the roots of the arrowroot plant and can be used as a substitute for cornstarch. You can find both in the baking aisle or where they sell the specialty grains and flours at most grocery stores, and they're readily available at health foods stores and online.

Per Serving: Calories: 245; Total Fat: 18g; Total Carbs: 20g; Fiber: 1g; Net Carbs: 19g; Protein: 3g

Onion Rings

Let's be honest: onion rings are absolutely amazing. They are crispy, savory, and oh-so-good. To make these AIP-friendly, the batter is made from a combination of cassava flour, coconut flour, and arrowroot starch. These are great served alone, or with Sticky Orange Wings (page 65) for a complete comfort food meal.

2 yellow onions, trimmed and peeled

4 to 6 cups avocado oil, or enough to fill a pot with 4 inches of oil

8 tablespoon cassava flour, divided

5 tablespoons arrowroot starch, divided

⅓ cup coconut flour

1 teaspoon pink Himalayan salt or sea salt

1¾ cups club soda

Ingredient Spotlight: We recommend using either a standard yellow onion or a white onion for these onion rings. For some reason, these seem to result in more crispy, tasty onion rings than other varieties.

1. Slice the onions about ¼ inch thick, and separate the rings.

2. Pour the avocado oil in a large pot over high heat and heat to 365°F. To see if it's hot enough, stick the handle of a wooden spoon into the oil. You should see bubbles form around the wood and start to float up.

3. In a small bowl, combine 2 tablespoons of cassava flour and 2 tablespoons of arrowroot starch. Dust the onion rings with the flour mixture.

4. In a medium bowl, combine the remaining 6 tablespoons cassava flour, remaining 3 tablespoons arrowroot starch, coconut flour, salt, and club soda, and whisk until combined.

5. Dip the onion rings one at a time into the batter and then carefully place in the hot oil, being careful not to overcrowd the rings (we recommend only 3 to 4 at a time). Fry for 3 to 4 minutes, or until golden brown, turning as needed.

6. Transfer the fried onion rings to a wire rack to cool slightly. Serve hot.

7. Store any leftovers in an airtight container in the refrigerator for up to 3 days (but these are best eaten right away).

Per Serving: Calories: 227; Total Fat: 16g; Total Carbs: 17g; Fiber: 4g; Net Carbs: 13g; Protein: 6g

Oven-Fried Chicken Nuggets

SERVES 4 / PREP TIME: 10 MINUTES
MARINATE TIME: 10 MINUTES / COOK TIME: 20 MINUTES

These Oven-Fried Chicken Nuggets will soon be a staple in your home, as both kids and adults love them. We bake these nuggets to ensure they are perfectly tender and crisp every single time. They taste great on their own, or you can serve them with AIP Barbecue Sauce (page 186).

½ cup full-fat unsweetened coconut milk (store-bought or homemade, page 174)

1 tablespoon white wine vinegar

½ teaspoon pink Himalayan salt or sea salt

1 pound boneless, skinless chicken breasts, cut into 1½-inch pieces

1½ cups crushed plain pork rinds

1. Preheat the oven to 400°F. Line a large baking sheet with parchment paper.

2. In a large baking pan, mix together the coconut milk, vinegar, and salt. Add the chicken pieces and let sit for 10 minutes.

3. Pour the pork rinds into a shallow bowl. One at a time, remove the chicken pieces from the baking pan, let the excess coconut milk mixture drip off, and coat in the pork rinds, firmly pressing the crumbs onto the chicken.

4. Place on the lined baking sheet in a single layer and bake for 16 to 20 minutes, or until crisp and golden brown. Serve hot.

5. Store any leftovers in an airtight container in the refrigerator for up to 3 to 4 days (but these are best eaten right away).

Ingredient Spotlight: Pork rinds, also known as chicharrones or cracklins, are made by cooking the skin of pigs until it's light and crispy. They can be found online or at the local grocery store in the chip aisle. Check the label and make sure there are no additives or non-AIP spices.

Per Serving: Calories: 238; Total Fat: 12g; Total Carbs: 1g; Fiber: 0g; Net Carbs: 1g; Protein: 31g

Sticky Orange Wings

SERVES 4 / PREP TIME: 10 MINUTES / COOK TIME: 40 MINUTES

Looking for an easy game-day appetizer that the whole crowd will love? Look no further! All you have to do is throw these wings in the oven and make a quick wing sauce while they are baking. With hints of sweet citrus, these wings are finger-licking good.

20 precut chicken wings (drumettes, winglets, or a combination of both)

1 tablespoon orange zest

Juice of 1 orange

2 garlic cloves, minced

1 tablespoon avocado oil

1 tablespoon red wine vinegar

2 tablespoons coconut aminos

2 scallions, chopped (optional)

1. Preheat the oven to 450°F.

2. Pat the wings dry with paper towels and place them on a large baking sheet. Bake for 30 to 40 minutes, or until the internal temperature reaches 165°F.

3. While the wings are baking, prepare the sauce by combining the orange zest, orange juice, garlic, avocado oil, vinegar, and coconut aminos in a small saucepan over medium heat. Cook until the sauce starts bubbling, then reduce the heat and simmer for 15 minutes, or until thickened.

4. Transfer the cooked wings to a bowl and pour the sauce over them. Toss to coat.

5. Plate the wings and garnish them with the chopped scallions, if using. Serve hot.

6. Store any leftovers in an airtight container in the refrigerator for up to 3 to 4 days.

Ingredient Spotlight: If you can't find precut wings, just buy whole wings and cut them at the joints to separate the drums and flats; discard the tips. Use a meat thermometer to ensure the chicken has reached 165°F before serving.

Per Serving: Calories: 329; Total Fat: 20g; Total Carbs: 3g; Fiber: 0g; Net Carbs: 3g; Protein: 24g

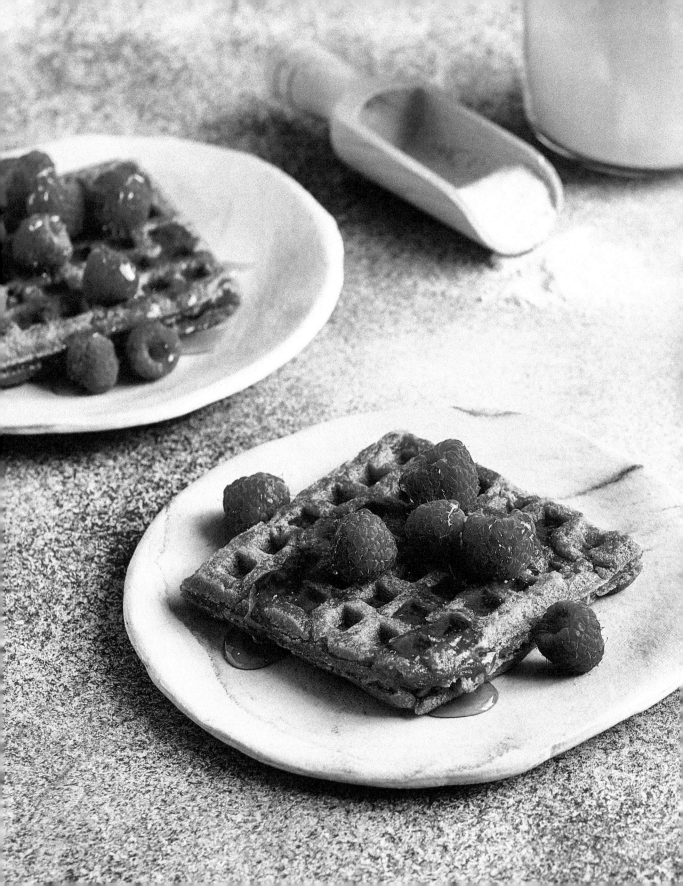

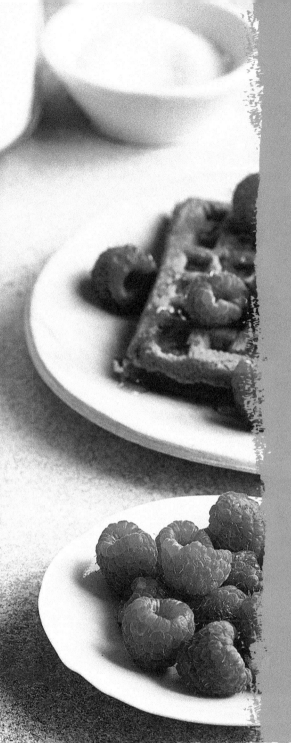

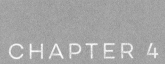

CHAPTER 4

BREAKFASTS

Pumpkin Waffles page 78

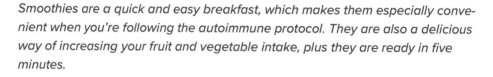

Green Goddess Smoothie

SERVES 1 / PREP TIME: 5 MINUTES

Smoothies are a quick and easy breakfast, which makes them especially convenient when you're following the autoimmune protocol. They are also a delicious way of increasing your fruit and vegetable intake, plus they are ready in five minutes.

1 cup baby spinach

½ avocado

2 kiwis, peeled

½ banana

½ cup full-fat unsweetened coconut milk (store-bought or homemade, page 174)

1. Put the spinach, avocado, kiwi, banana, and coconut milk in a blender and process until smooth.

2. Pour into a glass and enjoy. Smoothies are best when you drink them right away.

Ingredient Spotlight: A great way to tell that an avocado is ripe is to remove the little stem cap. If it comes off easily and is green underneath, you know you've got a ripe avocado that is ready to eat. If it's brown underneath, it's overripe.

Per Serving: Calories: 548; Total Fat: 41g; Total Carbs: 50g; Fiber: 15g; Net Carbs: 35g; Protein: 9g

Pumpkin Spice Smoothie

SERVES 1 / PREP TIME: 5 MINUTES

This frozen smoothie has the feel of fall and features warming autumn flavors like pumpkin and cinnamon. Pumpkin is rich in vitamin A, beta-carotene, iron, B vitamins, folate, phosphorus, and magnesium, making it a wonderful AIP-compliant food. If you buy canned pumpkin, make sure you get plain 100-percent pumpkin puree and not pumpkin pie filling, which has added sugar and spices.

½ cup pumpkin puree

½ banana

½ cup full-fat unsweetened coconut milk (store-bought or homemade, page 174)

½ teaspoon cinnamon

Pinch ground ginger

1 teaspoon pure maple syrup

1 cup ice

1. Combine the pumpkin, banana, coconut milk, cinnamon, ginger, maple syrup, and ice in a blender and process until smooth.

2. Pour into a glass and enjoy. Smoothies are best when you drink them right away.

Ingredient Spotlight: Don't be fooled by imitation maple syrups at the grocery store. Make sure the label says 100-percent pure maple syrup and the only ingredient is pure organic maple syrup. The darker the maple syrup, the stronger and more robust the flavor will be. Many people prefer a medium-dark amber syrup.

Per Serving: Calories: 337; Total Fat: 25g; Total Carbs: 32g; Fiber: 6g; Net Carbs: 26g; Protein: 4g

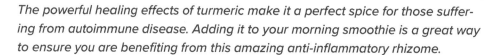

Coconut Turmeric Smoothie

SERVES 1 / PREP TIME: 5 MINUTES

The powerful healing effects of turmeric make it a perfect spice for those suffering from autoimmune disease. Adding it to your morning smoothie is a great way to ensure you are benefiting from this amazing anti-inflammatory rhizome.

½ cup full-fat unsweetened coconut milk (store-bought or homemade, page 174)

¼ cup plain unsweetened coconut yogurt

1 banana

1 teaspoon ground turmeric

1 tablespoon raw honey

¼ cup filtered water

1. Put the coconut milk, coconut yogurt, banana, turmeric, honey, and water in a blender and process until smooth.

2. Pour into a glass and enjoy. Smoothies are best when you drink them right away.

Swap or Substitute: For a bigger breakfast, pour the smoothie into a bowl and top it with our On-the-Go Granola (page 75). For a more filling smoothie, add 1 tablespoon of unflavored collagen powder.

Per Serving: Calories: 438; Total Fat: 27g; Total Carbs: 52g; Fiber: 4g; Net Carbs: 48g; Protein: 6g

Tropical Pineapple Smoothie

SERVES 1 / PREP TIME: 5 MINUTES

Frozen pineapple and mango give this smoothie a tropical flavor. Pineapples contain digestive enzymes called bromelain, which help break down protein molecules so they are easier for the small intestine to absorb.

1 cup frozen
pineapple chunks

½ banana

¼ cup frozen
mango chunks

½ cup orange juice

½ cup full-fat unsweetened
coconut milk (store-bought
or homemade, page 174)

1. Combine the pineapple, banana, mango, orange juice, and coconut milk in a blender and process until smooth.

2. Pour into a glass and enjoy. Smoothies are best when you drink them right away.

Ingredient Spotlight: Frozen fruit is perfect to use in smoothies. It is cheaper, can be stored longer, and is picked at the peak of ripeness.

Per Serving: Calories: 438; Total Fat: 25g; Total Carbs: 57g; Fiber: 5g; Net Carbs: 52g; Protein: 5g

Cinnamon Apple Smoothie

SERVES 1 / PREP TIME: 5 MINUTES

The tart apples in this tasty smoothie are balanced perfectly with warm cinnamon notes. Any variety of apple will work with this recipe, so feel free to use your favorite.

1 apple, cored and roughly chopped

½ banana

½ cup full-fat unsweetened coconut milk (store-bought or homemade, page 174)

½ teaspoon cinnamon

½ teaspoon vanilla powder

1 cup ice

1. Put the apple, banana, coconut milk, cinnamon, vanilla powder, and ice in a blender and process until smooth.

2. Pour into a glass and enjoy. Smoothies are best when you drink them right away.

Swap or Substitute: For a more filling breakfast, add a scoop of unflavored collagen peptides to the blender; they're packed with protein and amino acids.

Per Serving: Calories: 373; Total Fat: 25g; Total Carbs: 43g; Fiber: 7g; Net Carbs: 36g; Protein: 3g

Berry and Kale Smoothie

This smoothie cleverly sneaks kale into your breakfast so you can start your day off right. We also use blackberries and blueberries to give this delicious frozen drink a gorgeous dark purple color.

1 cup torn lacinato kale leaves, stems removed

½ cup blackberries

½ cup blueberries

½ banana

½ cup full-fat unsweetened coconut milk (store-bought or homemade, page 174)

1 tablespoon collagen peptides powder

1 cup ice

1. Combine the kale, blackberries, blueberries, banana, coconut milk, collagen powder, and ice in a blender and process until smooth.

2. Pour into a glass and enjoy. Smoothies are best when you drink them right away.

Ingredient Spotlight: If your produce tends to go bad before you finish eating all of it, try buying frozen blueberries and blackberries. They will work perfectly in this smoothie and last much longer than fresh berries.

Per Serving: Calories: 391; Total Fat: 25g; Total Carbs: 36g; Fiber: 8g; Net Carbs: 28g; Protein: 14g

Strawberry Coconut Parfait

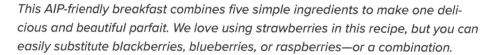

SERVES 1 / PREP TIME: 5 MINUTES

This AIP-friendly breakfast combines five simple ingredients to make one delicious and beautiful parfait. We love using strawberries in this recipe, but you can easily substitute blackberries, blueberries, or raspberries—or a combination.

1 cup plain unsweetened coconut yogurt

1 tablespoon raw honey

½ teaspoon vanilla powder

1 cup chopped strawberries

½ cup On-the-Go Granola (page 75)

1. In a small bowl, mix together the coconut yogurt, honey, and vanilla powder until combined.

2. In a large glass, spoon one-third of the yogurt mixture into the bottom, followed by one-third of the strawberries, then one-third of the granola. Repeat the same layers twice more.

3. Serve immediately.

4. If you're making extra parfaits, store the yogurt and the granola separately and put the parfait together right before serving, so the granola will not get soggy.

Swap or Substitute: Feel free to swap frozen strawberries for the fresh ones. Just thaw them for 5 to 10 minutes before using.

Per Serving: Calories: 423; Total Fat: 18g; Total Carbs: 67g; Fiber: 11g; Net Carbs: 56g; Protein: 2g

On-the-Go Granola

This granola is our AIP-friendly version of those store-bought cereals that are full of grains and added sugar. The sweetness in this granola comes naturally from the coconut and dried fruit. You will never go back to the store-bought stuff after trying this recipe.

2 cups coconut flakes, lightly crushed

1 cup Baked Cinnamon Apple Chips (page 52), lightly crushed

½ cup plantain chips, lightly crushed

½ cup dried blueberries

2 teaspoons cinnamon

2 tablespoons coconut oil, melted

2 tablespoons raw honey

1. Preheat the oven to 325°F. Line a large baking sheet with parchment paper.

2. In a large bowl, gently mix together the coconut flakes, apple chips, plantain chips, dried blueberries, cinnamon, coconut oil, and honey.

3. Spread the mixture on the baking sheet in an even layer and bake for 10 to 15 minutes, stirring halfway. The mixture can burn easily, so keep an eye on it.

4. Allow the granola to cool completely before enjoying alone or with full-fat unsweetened coconut milk, with plain unsweetened coconut yogurt, or on top of a smoothie.

5. Store leftovers in an airtight container at room temperature for up to 7 days.

Ingredient Spotlight: Plantains are a member of the banana family, and while they look very similar to bananas, they are more starchy and less sweet. Plantains are a good source of potassium, magnesium, and vitamins A, C, and B6. Look for plantain chips that are cooked in coconut oil. We like Banana Organic or Terra plantain chips. Or you can make your own in 20 minutes by peeling and thinly slicing a green plantain, then frying the slices with coconut oil in a sturdy skillet. Cook the plantain slices just until they start to turn slightly brown, and then transfer them to a plate lined with paper towels. Let them cool completely before using in this recipe.

Per Serving: Calories: 446; Total Fat: 25g; Total Carbs: 60g; Fiber: 10g; Net Carbs: 50g; Protein: 2g

Honey Spiced "Noatmeal"

This breakfast is so warm, comforting, and versatile. You'll be so surprised that cauliflower makes the perfect oatmeal replacement! Eat as is, or top with any dried fruit of your choice, such as blueberries, dates, or apricots.

¾ cups full-fat unsweetened coconut milk (store-bought or homemade, page 174)

¼ cup shredded coconut

¼ cup cauliflower rice, fresh or frozen

1 banana, mashed

⅛ teaspoon pink Himalayan salt or sea salt

½ teaspoon gluten-free vanilla extract

½ tablespoon raw honey

1. Combine the coconut milk, shredded coconut, cauliflower rice, and banana in a large pot over low heat. Bring to a simmer, then cook for 15 minutes.

2. Stir in the salt and vanilla extract and simmer for an additional 5 minutes.

3. Transfer the "Noatmeal" to bowls and drizzle with the honey. Serve warm. This is best enjoyed right away.

Make It Easier: Having a big bag of cauliflower rice in the freezer is a great way to make sure you always have some on hand without worrying about it going bad.

Per Serving: Calories: 277; Total Fat: 22g; Total Carbs: 23g; Fiber: 3g; Net Carbs: 20g; Protein: 3g

Banana Pancakes

Bananas provide just a touch of sweetness to these fluffy pancakes that come together in only 20 minutes. Just combine all the ingredients in a blender for an easy and delicious meal. Make a double batch and freeze the extra pancakes for an easy weekday breakfast. Simply reheat them for 5 minutes in a 350°F oven.

2 bananas

⅓ cup cassava flour

⅓ cup tigernut flour

1 teaspoon baking soda

½ teaspoon pink Himalayan salt or sea salt

2½ tablespoons coconut oil, melted

2½ tablespoons filtered water

2 teaspoons cinnamon

1. Combine the bananas, cassava flour, tigernut flour, baking soda, salt, coconut oil, water, and cinnamon in a blender and pulse until smooth.

2. Heat a skillet over medium-low heat. Pour the batter into the skillet to form 4-inch circles. Cook for about 2 minutes. When the bottoms are golden brown and bubbles have formed on the tops, flip the pancakes and cook for about 2 minutes more.

3. Serve warm.

4. Store any leftovers in an airtight container in the refrigerator for up to 5 days or in the freezer for up to 3 months.

Ingredient Spotlight: Tigernut flour is made from ground tigernuts, which are small tubers that are native to Africa. They're a great source of vitamins E, C, and B₆, as well as resistant starch, which is a prebiotic that helps the good bacteria grow in the intestines. You can find the flour in health food stores or you can order it online.

Per Serving: Calories: 197; Total Fat: 10g; Total Carbs: 27g; Fiber: 4g; Net Carbs: 23g; Protein: 3g

Pumpkin Waffles

So comforting and warming, these healthy pumpkin waffles are perfect for when you want something that will fill you up all morning long. To make this dish completely AIP-friendly, make sure to use aluminum-free baking powder. Make a double batch and freeze the extra waffles so you have them ready to eat throughout the week. Just reheat them for 5 minutes in a 350°F oven for a quick breakfast. You can top these waffles with fresh fruit, like raspberries or strawberries, if desired.

1½ cups cassava flour

½ cup tigernut flour

½ cup pumpkin puree

¼ cup coconut sugar

1 teaspoon baking powder

½ teaspoon baking soda

½ cup coconut oil, melted

2 tablespoons beef gelatin powder

1 teaspoon gluten-free vanilla extract

½ teaspoon pink Himalayan salt or sea salt

1. Combine the cassava flour, tigernut flour, pumpkin puree, coconut sugar, baking powder, baking soda, coconut oil, beef gelatin powder, vanilla extract, and salt in a blender and pulse until smooth. If the batter is too thick, add filtered water one tablespoon at a time until pourable.

2. Heat a waffle iron to high heat. Pour all the batter into the hot waffle iron and close the lid. (Most waffle irons make four waffles at a time. If yours doesn't, you will need to repeat this step accordingly to yield four waffles.)

3. When the waffle iron indicates that the waffles are done, remove and serve while they are still hot. Top with pure maple syrup or raw honey, if desired.

4. Store any leftovers in an airtight container in the refrigerator for up to 5 days or in the freezer up to 3 months.

Ingredient Spotlight: Beef gelatin powder can be used as a binding agent in AIP baking. It is perfect for replacing an egg in baked recipes, as it has the ability to hold ingredients together and prevent food from crumbling or falling apart.

Per Serving: Calories: 527; Total Fat: 28g; Total Carbs: 63g; Fiber: 7g; Net Carbs: 56g; Protein: 10g

Cinnamon Zucchini Muffins

MAKES 8 / PREP TIME: 10 MINUTES / COOK TIME: 25 MINUTES

The zucchini in these muffins give them an incredibly moist and chewy texture. Zucchini is a rich source of B vitamins, including folate, riboflavin, and B6, which can help boost energy production in the body and can ease the fatigue that people with autoimmune disease often experience. Feel free to increase this recipe so you have extra muffins on hand to enjoy throughout the week as a quick breakfast or snack.

1 cup tigernut flour

¼ cup cassava flour

2 tablespoons coconut flour

1 cup shredded zucchini

½ teaspoon baking soda

2 teaspoons cinnamon

¼ cup pure maple syrup

2 tablespoons coconut sugar

6 tablespoons coconut oil, melted

2 Gelatin Eggs (page 187)

1. Preheat the oven to 375°F. Line 8 cups of a muffin tin with cupcake liners.

2. In a large bowl, combine the tigernut flour, cassava flour, coconut flour, zucchini, baking soda, cinnamon, maple syrup, coconut sugar, and coconut oil. Stir in the gelatin eggs until they are completely combined.

3. Spoon the batter into the muffin liners and bake for 22 to 25 minutes, or until the muffins are cooked through the center.

4. Cool the muffins in the tin before eating.

5. Store any leftover muffins in an airtight container at room temperature for up to 5 days or in the freezer for up to 3 months.

Make It Easier: To check whether the muffins are cooked through, insert a toothpick into the center of one. If it comes out clean and without any wet batter attached, you know the muffins are done.

Per Serving: Calories: 200; Total Fat: 12g; Total Carbs: 20g; Fiber: 5g; Net Carbs: 15g; Protein: 3g

Carrot Cake Muffins

MAKES: 8 MUFFINS / PREP TIME: 10 MINUTES / COOK TIME: 25 MINUTES

No one will know that this delicious breakfast muffin is made with all healthy and anti-inflammatory ingredients. Carrots are a rich source of vitamin C, which can activate the white blood cells in your body. Make these muffins to serve at a weekend brunch, or take them with you for an on-the-go breakfast.

1 cup tigernut flour

¼ cup cassava flour

2 tablespoons coconut flour

1 cup shredded carrots

½ teaspoon baking soda

2 teaspoons cinnamon

¼ cup pure maple syrup

2 tablespoons coconut sugar

6 tablespoons coconut oil, melted

2 Gelatin Eggs (page 187)

1. Preheat the oven to 375 °F. Line 8 cups of a muffin tin with cupcake liners.

2. In a large bowl, combine the tigernut flour, cassava flour, coconut flour, carrots, baking soda, cinnamon, maple syrup, coconut sugar, and coconut oil. Stir in the gelatin eggs until completely combined.

3. Spoon the batter into the muffin liners and bake for 22 to 25 minutes, or until the muffins are cooked through the center and a toothpick inserted into one comes out clean.

4. Cool the muffins in the tin before eating.

5. Store any leftovers in an airtight container at room temperature for up to 5 days or in the freezer for up to 3 months.

Make It Easier: Save yourself some time and buy shredded carrots at the supermarket. You'll find them with the other produce.

Per Serving: Calories: 175; Total Fat: 12g; Total Carbs: 19g; Fiber: 14g; Net Carbs: 5g; Protein: 3g

Raspberry Breakfast Bars

MAKES 12 BARS / PREP TIME: 5 MINUTES / COOK TIME: 20 MINUTES

These breakfast bars are a delicious and noninflammatory way to start your day. This recipe makes 12 bars, so make a batch on the weekend and you and your family will have an easy breakfast option for the whole week. Or freeze the extra bars and take them out when you need them.

1 cup tigernut flour

¼ cup cassava flour

2 tablespoons collagen peptides powder

½ banana, mashed

½ teaspoon baking soda

2 teaspoons cinnamon

¼ cup pure maple syrup

2 tablespoons coconut sugar

6 tablespoons coconut oil, melted

2 Gelatin Eggs (page 187)

1 cup fresh raspberries

1. Preheat the oven to 350°F. Line an 8-by-11-inch baking pan with parchment paper.

2. In a large bowl, mix together the tigernut flour, cassava flour, collagen powder, banana, baking soda, cinnamon, maple syrup, coconut sugar, and coconut oil until combined. Immediately stir in the gelatin eggs. Fold in the raspberries.

3. Transfer the mixture to the baking pan and use a spatula to spread it out evenly. Bake for 16 to 20 minutes, or until it's cooked through and golden brown.

4. Allow the mixture to fully cool in the pan before cutting into 12 bars.

5. Store extra bars in an airtight container at room temperature for up to 5 days or in the freezer for up to 3 months.

Swap or Substitute: The raspberries can be swapped out for the berry of your choice, such as strawberries, blue-berries, or blackberries. You can also use frozen berries; just let them thaw for 10 minutes before adding them to the batter.

Per Serving: Calories: 160; Total Fat: 9g; Total Carbs: 18g; Fiber: 4g; Net Carbs: 14g; Protein: 1g

Smoked Salmon with Avocado

Loaded with healthy fats, this breakfast is simple, savory, and will keep you satisfied until lunch. And for a delicious variation, put all the ingredients on top of our AIP Garlic Herb Flatbread (page 62). If you don't have time to make AIP Mayo (page 179), drizzle extra-virgin olive oil over top of the salmon instead.

1 avocado, pitted, peeled, and sliced

2 tablespoons AIP Mayo (page 179)

8 ounces smoked salmon

1 tablespoon capers

1 tablespoon chopped fresh dill (optional)

1. Divide the avocado slices between two medium plates, then add a dollop of mayo and half the salmon, capers, and dill (if using) to each plate.

2. Enjoy immediately.

Swap or Substitute: Not a fan of smoked salmon? You can swap it for tuna in a can or cooked shrimp.

Per Serving: Calories: 436; Total Fat: 34g; Total Carbs: 12g; Fiber: 9g; Net Carbs: 3g; Protein: 24g

Open-Face Breakfast Sandwich

SERVES 2 / PREP TIME: 10 MINUTES / COOK TIME: 20 MINUTES

This fresh and savory sandwich is the perfect way to incorporate healthy arugula and avocado into your breakfast. Make a batch of AIP Garlic Herb Flatbread (page 62) and some AIP Mayo (page 179) ahead of time, so all you need to do is fry up some bacon and assemble.

6 slices bacon

2 tablespoons AIP Mayo (page 179)

2 AIP Garlic Herb Flatbreads (page 62)

½ cup arugula

½ avocado, peeled, pitted, and sliced

1. In a large skillet, cook the bacon over medium heat for 10 to 12 minutes, or until it's crisp. Transfer to a plate lined with paper towels.

2. Lay out the flatbreads, and spread 1 tablespoon of mayo on each one. Divide the arugula between the flatbreads, then top with 3 bacon slices. Arrange the avocado on top of the bacon.

3. Enjoy right away.

Make It Easier: For an easy and quick assembly, make the bacon, flatbread, and mayo ahead of time; they'll keep in the refrigerator for up to 3 to 4 days. You'll be able to enjoy this sandwich whenever you get the craving.

Per Serving: Calories: 619; Total Fat: 52g; Total Carbs: 27g; Fiber: 5g; Net Carbs: 22g; Protein: 16g

Sweet Potato Hash

SERVES 4 / PREP TIME: 5 MINUTES / COOK TIME: 25 MINUTES

This simple and satisfying breakfast can be ready to serve in 30 minutes. Sweet potatoes are high in fiber and antioxidants that can aid in digestive health. This recipe is perfect for reheating as leftovers, so make a double batch and enjoy it throughout the week.

2 tablespoons avocado oil

1 yellow onion, diced

2 garlic cloves, minced

2 large sweet potatoes, peeled and diced small

1 pound pork sausage or ground pork

1 teaspoon pink Himalayan salt or sea salt

2 tablespoons pure maple syrup

½ teaspoon dried thyme or 1 teaspoon chopped fresh thyme

1. Heat the avocado oil in a large skillet over medium-high heat, then add the onion and garlic. Sauté, stirring constantly, until softened, about 5 minutes. Add the sweet potatoes and cook for another 5 minutes. Add the pork and cook, using a spatula to crumble it, until cooked through and browned, 5 to 8 minutes.

2. Add the salt, maple syrup, and thyme and cook for 5 more minutes.

3. Serve hot.

4. Store any leftovers in an airtight container in the refrigerator for up to 3 to 4 days.

Ingredient Spotlight: Make sure to check the pork sausage label to ensure the spices are AIP-friendly. You are looking for no sugar, no black pepper, and no other non-AIP spices listed on page 14. You can also make your own sausage using the recipe in Homemade Biscuits and Sausage Gravy (page 86), or just use plain ground pork.

Per Serving: Calories: 294; Total Fat: 12g; Total Carbs: 23g; Fiber: 3g; Net Carbs: 20g; Protein: 25g

Breakfast Sausage Casserole

SERVES 4 / PREP TIME: 5 MINUTES / COOK TIME: 30 MINUTES

Parsnips are rich in antioxidants, fiber, folate, and vitamin K. When cooked their flavor is a bit sweet, and the texture is a cross between a potato and a carrot, making them the perfect base for a hearty casserole. This one features all your breakfast favorites in a single dish.

6 parsnips, peeled and roughly chopped

2 tablespoons avocado oil

1 yellow onion, diced

2 garlic cloves, minced

1 pound pork sausage or ground pork

1 teaspoon pink Himalayan salt or sea salt, divided

½ teaspoon dried thyme or 2 teaspoons chopped fresh thyme, divided

¼ cup full-fat unsweetened coconut milk (store-bought or homemade, page 174)

6 slices bacon, cooked and chopped

Ingredient Spotlight: This casserole is a great way to use up any extra veggies you have in your refrigerator. After you cook the onion and garlic in step 3, add in cooked carrots, broccoli, spinach, or anything else you think would work.

1. Preheat the oven to 350°F.

2. Fill a large pot with 6 inches of filtered water, add the parsnips, and cover. Cook over high heat for about 15 minutes, or until the parsnips have softened.

3. While the parsnips are cooking, heat the avocado oil in a large ovenproof skillet over medium-high heat, and add the onion and garlic. Sauté, stirring constantly, until they are softened, about 5 minutes. Stir in the sausage, ½ teaspoon salt, and half the thyme. Cook, using a spatula to crumble the sausage, until cooked through and browned, 5 to 8 minutes.

4. When the parsnips are soft, drain them in a colander and transfer to a food processor or blender. Add the coconut milk, the remaining ½ teaspoon salt, and the remaining 1 teaspoon thyme. Pulse until combined. Transfer the mashed parsnips to the skillet with the pork mixture and stir until combined.

5. Top with the chopped bacon and put the skillet in the oven. Bake for about 15 minutes, or until heated through. Serve hot.

6. Store the leftovers in an airtight container in the refrigerator for up to 3 to 4 days.

Per Serving: Calories: 457; Total Fat: 20g; Total Carbs: 40g; Fiber: 10g; Net Carbs: 30g; Protein: 31g

Homemade Biscuits and Sausage Gravy

SERVES 4 / PREP TIME: 10 MINUTES / COOK TIME: 16 MINUTES

These biscuits with sausage gravy are comfort food made AIP-friendly at its finest. This savory and very hearty recipe freezes well, so go ahead and make a double or triple batch to have a quick breakfast on hand. Just make sure to store the biscuits and the sausage gravy in separate sealed containers in the freezer. Reheat in the oven at 350°F for 10 to 15 minutes, or until everything is heated through.

FOR THE BISCUITS

⅓ cup cassava flour

⅓ cup coconut flour

½ teaspoon baking soda

½ teaspoon pink Himalayan salt or sea salt

⅓ cup lard

¼ cup full-fat unsweetened coconut milk (store-bought or homemade, page 174)

½ teaspoon apple cider vinegar

1 tablespoon pure maple syrup

¼ teaspoon cream of tartar

3 Gelatin Eggs (page 187)

TO MAKE THE BISCUITS

1. Preheat the oven to 350°F. Line a large baking sheet with parchment paper.

2. In a medium bowl, combine the cassava flour, coconut flour, baking soda, and salt. Use a fork to mash the lard into the dry mixture. Stir in the coconut milk, apple cider vinegar, maple syrup, and cream of tartar. Mix in the gelatin eggs.

3. Divide the dough into 8 portions and place each portion on the lined baking sheet, gently forming them into biscuit shapes. Bake for 15 to 20 minutes, or until they start to brown on top.

1 pound ground pork

1 teaspoon dried sage

1 teaspoon pink Himalayan salt or sea salt

½ teaspoon dried thyme

½ teaspoon garlic powder

¼ teaspoon onion powder

2 tablespoons cassava flour

1 cup full-fat unsweetened coconut milk (store-bought or homemade, page 174)

TO MAKE THE SAUSAGE GRAVY

4. While the biscuits are baking, combine the pork, sage, salt, thyme, garlic powder, and onion powder in a large bowl.

5. Heat a large skillet over medium heat and brown the sausage, about 5 minutes. When it's cooked through, add the cassava flour and cook for 2 more minutes.

6. Stir in the coconut milk and let the gravy cook for 5 to 10 minutes more. Pour the sausage gravy over the biscuits to serve.

7. Store leftover gravy in an airtight container in the refrigerator for up to 3 to 4 days.

Make It Easier: These biscuits taste great on their own if you don't feel like making the sausage gravy. Top them with a little raw honey or pure maple syrup. Store any extra biscuits in an airtight container at room temperature for up to 3 to 4 days. You can also use this recipe to make your own pork sausage meat. Just combine everything as in step 1 for the sausage gravy, and you're done!

Per Serving: Calories: 558; Total Fat: 38g; Total Carbs: 24g; Fiber: 2g; Net Carbs: 22g; Protein: 34g

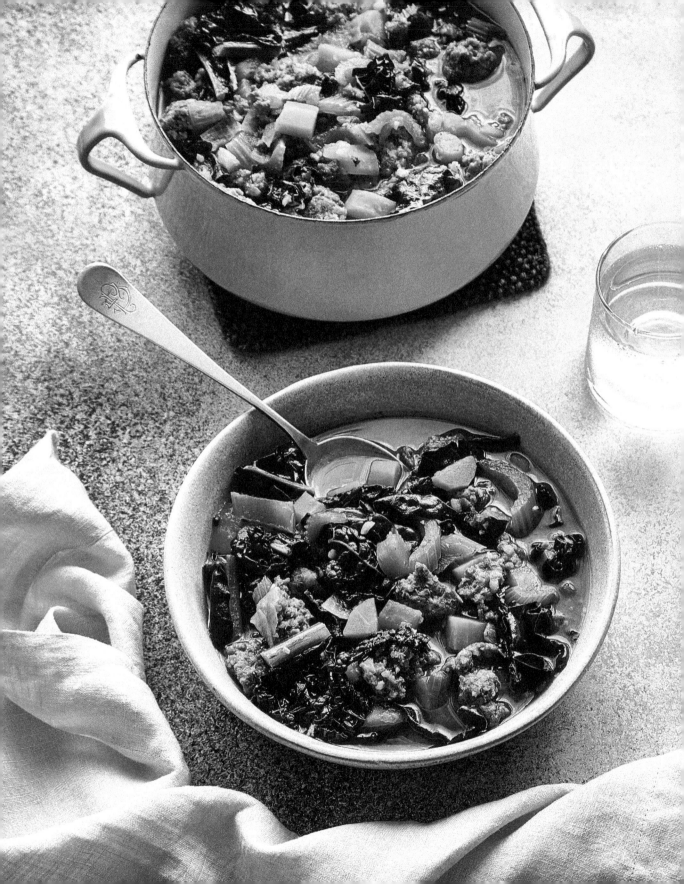

SOUPS AND SALADS

Tuscan Kale Soup *page 95*

Creamy Mushroom Soup

SERVES 4 / PREP TIME: 5 MINUTES / COOK TIME: 30 MINUTES

This soup is packed with flavor. The mushrooms provide an earthy savor, which contrasts perfectly with sweet caramelized shallots and creamy coconut milk. Plus, baby portobello mushrooms (also called criminis) contain micronutrients such as vitamin D, which is vital for immune function. If you have an immersion blender, use that directly in the soup pot to purée the soup until smooth.

2 tablespoons avocado oil

4 cups sliced baby portobello mushrooms

1 shallot, thinly sliced

4 garlic cloves, minced

6 cups Beef Bone Broth (store-bought or homemade, page 191)

3 sprigs fresh thyme

1 bay leaf

Pinch pink Himalayan salt or sea salt

1 cup full-fat unsweetened coconut milk (store-bought or homemade, page 174)

1. In a large pot, heat the avocado oil over medium heat. Add the mushrooms, shallot, and garlic, and sauté for about 10 minutes, until soft. Add the bone broth, thyme, bay leaf, and salt. Cover and simmer for 20 minutes.

2. Remove the bay leaf and thyme sprigs and stir in the coconut milk.

3. Working in batches, carefully transfer the soup to a blender and puree until smooth. Be extremely careful not to fill the blender too full of the hot soup, and cover the lid with a dish towel before you start blending.

4. Transfer to a soup bowl and enjoy.

5. Store any leftovers in an airtight container in the refrigerator for up to 3 to 4 days.

Swap or Substitute: You can use white button mushrooms instead of baby portobellos, or a combination of both.

Per Serving: Calories: 238; Total Fat: 19g; Total Carbs: 7g; Fiber: 0g; Net Carbs: 7g; Protein: 12g

Butternut Squash Soup

SERVES 4 / PREP TIME: 5 MINUTES / COOK TIME: 35 MINUTES

Butternut squash is the perfect base for a warm, creamy, delicious soup. This winter squash has gorgeous orange flesh and is packed with vitamins A and C. Roasting the butternut squash in the oven caramelizes it and really brings out the sweet and nutty flavor.

1 medium (about 3 pounds) butternut squash, peeled, seeded, and diced

1 white onion, chopped into 1-inch pieces

4 garlic cloves, minced

¼ cup avocado oil

Pinch pink Himalayan salt or sea salt

3 cups Chicken Bone Broth (store-bought or homemade, page 190)

1 cup full-fat unsweetened coconut milk (store-bought or homemade, page 174)

1 teaspoon cinnamon

Make It Easier: To save time, buy precut butternut squash if you can find it at your local grocery store. If you have an immersion blender, use that directly in the soup pot to puree the soup until smooth.

1. Preheat the oven to 400°F. Line a large baking sheet with parchment paper.

2. Put the butternut squash, onion, and garlic on the sheet, toss with the avocado oil, and season liberally with salt. Roast for 25 to 30 minutes, until tender.

3. While the vegetables are roasting, pour the bone broth into a large pot and bring to a boil. Turn down the heat and simmer. Add the roasted vegetables and simmer for 5 more minutes.

4. Working in batches, carefully transfer the soup to a blender and puree. Be extremely careful not to fill the blender too full of the hot soup and cover the lid with a dish towel before you start blending.

5. Pour the pureed soup back into the pot and stir in the coconut milk and cinnamon. Taste and season with more salt, if needed. If the soup is too thick, whisk in additional bone broth until you've reached the desired consistency. Serve warm.

6. Store in the refrigerator for up to 3 to 4 days or freeze for up to 3 months.

Per Serving: Calories: 424; Total Fat: 26g; Total Carbs: 43g; Fiber: 6g; Net Carbs: 37g; Protein: 11g

French Onion Soup

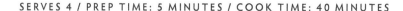

SERVES 4 / PREP TIME: 5 MINUTES / COOK TIME: 40 MINUTES

The secret to a good French onion soup is making sure you caramelize the onions. Rather than browning them, you want to cook them low and slow so that the natural sugars create a wonderful flavor. This soups pairs perfectly with the biscuits from our Homemade Biscuits and Sausage Gravy (page 86) recipe.

¼ cup avocado oil

4 yellow onions, thinly sliced (4 to 5 cups)

2 bay leaves

2 sprigs fresh thyme

1 teaspoon coconut sugar

2 tablespoons arrowroot starch

6 cups Beef Bone Broth (store-bought or homemade, page 191)

Pinch pink Himalayan salt or sea salt

1. In a large pot, heat the avocado oil over medium heat. Add the onions, bay leaves, thyme, and coconut sugar, and sauté for about 5 minutes, until soft. Turn down the heat to low, cover, and let the onions cook for 20 more minutes to fully caramelized, stirring occasionally.

2. Sprinkle the arrowroot starch over the onions and slowly whisk in the bone broth. Cover and simmer for 20 minutes.

3. Remove the bay leaves and thyme sprigs and season with salt. Enjoy warm.

4. Store any leftovers in an airtight container in the refrigerator for up to 3 to 4 days.

Swap or Substitute: You can use white onions instead of the yellow onions, or use a combination of both. For caramelized onions, it's best to slice them lengthwise from stem to root so that the onions slices hold their shape better.

Per Serving: Calories: 203; Total Fat: 14g; Total Carbs: 6g; Fiber: 0g; Net Carbs: 6g; Protein: 15g

Thai Shrimp Soup

SERVES 4 / PREP TIME: 5 MINUTES / COOK TIME: 45 MINUTES

Skip the takeout and make this Thai-inspired soup at home. It's unbelievably tasty and super simple to make. This soup is aromatic and flavorful, thanks to all the classic Thai ingredients, including ginger, red curry, fish sauce, and lime. Bruising the lemongrass and ginger helps release their oils and flavors, so don't skip this step.

1 stalk fresh lemongrass, outer layers removed

1-inch piece fresh ginger, peeled

4 cups Chicken Bone Broth (store-bought or homemade, page 190)

Zest of 1 lime

2 tablespoons lime juice

1 cup stemmed shiitake mushrooms

1 pound shrimp, peeled and deveined

1 cup full-fat unsweetened coconut milk (store-bought or homemade, page 174)

1 tablespoon fish sauce

1 teaspoon raw honey

2 tablespoons finely chopped fresh cilantro

1. With the back of a knife, lightly smash the lemongrass and ginger. Cut the lemongrass into 4-inch pieces.

2. In a large pot, bring the lemongrass, ginger, bone broth, lime zest. and lime juice to a boil, then reduce the heat to low and simmer for 10 minutes. Use a slotted spoon to remove the lemongrass and ginger pieces from the soup and skim off any other particles that float to the top.

3. Add the mushrooms. Cook for 25 minutes, then stir in the shrimp, coconut milk, fish sauce, honey, and cilantro. Cook for 2 to 3 more minutes, making sure not to overcook the shrimp. Serve immediately.

4. Serve immediately.

5. Store any leftovers in an airtight container in the refrigerator for up to 3 to 4 days.

Ingredient Spotlight: Fish sauce is a liquid condiment made from fish that has been coated in salt and fermented— and trust us, it tastes a lot better than it sounds! If you don't have fish sauce, you can substitute coconut aminos.

Per Serving: Calories: 246; Total Fat: 13g; Total Carbs: 6g; Fiber: 0g; Net Carbs: 6g; Protein: 27g

Immune-Boosting Chicken Soup

SERVES 4 / PREP TIME: 5 MINUTES / COOK TIME: 30 MINUTES

Our AIP version of this classic soup is loaded with immune-boosting powerhouses like ginger, garlic, turmeric, and bone broth, which work in perfect harmony to help the body heal and recover. Enjoy it often to get all its amazing benefits.

4 tablespoons avocado oil

½ cup celery, chopped into ½-inch pieces

½ cup yellow onion, chopped into ½-inch pieces

¼ cup carrots, chopped into ½-inch pieces

2 garlic cloves, minced

6 cups Chicken Bone Broth (store-bought or homemade, page 190)

2 teaspoons ground turmeric

1 teaspoon curry powder

1 teaspoon grated fresh ginger

1 teaspoon pink Himalayan salt or sea salt

8 boneless, skinless chicken thighs

1 cup full-fat unsweetened coconut milk (store-bought or homemade, page 174)

1. In a large pot, heat the avocado oil over medium heat. Add the celery, onion, and carrot, and sauté for about 4 minutes, until soft. Add the garlic and sauté for an additional 1 minute.

2. Add the bone broth, turmeric, curry powder, ginger, salt, and chicken thighs. Bring to a boil, then cover and reduce the heat to low. Simmer for 10 to 15 minutes, or until the chicken is cooked through.

3. Remove the chicken and let it cool for 5 minutes. Use two forks to shred it.

4. Whisk the coconut milk into the soup. Return the shredded chicken to the soup and stir to combine. Simmer for 5 more minutes. Serve immediately.

5. Store any leftover soup in an airtight container in the refrigerator for up to 3 to 4 days or in the freezer for up to 3 months.

Make It Easier: Look for pre-cut onions, carrots, and celery in the produce section of the grocery store. Also, if you have a batch of Shredded Chicken (page 188) already cooked, use that instead of the chicken thighs in this recipe. Just add it in step 4.

Per Serving: Calories: 633; Total Fat: 38g; Total Carbs: 6g; Fiber: 1g; Net Carbs: 5g; Protein: 65g

Tuscan Kale Soup

SERVES 4 / PREP TIME: 5 MINUTES / COOK TIME: 30 MINUTES

Also known as Zuppa Toscana, this hearty soup originates from the Tuscany region of Italy. Tuscany is known for its simple and efficient cuisine, and especially for its tradition of making soup. We have put our own AIP spin on this one by loading it with nutrient-dense vegetables and flavorful pork to create a hearty and healthy one-pot meal.

2 tablespoons avocado oil

1 yellow onion, chopped into ½-inch pieces

3 celery stalks, chopped into ½-inch pieces

3 carrots, chopped into ½-inch pieces

4 garlic cloves, minced

1 teaspoon pink Himalayan salt or sea salt

2 teaspoons dried oregano

1½ pounds pork sausage or ground pork

6 cups Chicken Bone Broth (store-bought or homemade, page 190)

1 cup coarsely chopped lacinato kale

1. Heat the avocado oil in a large pot over medium-high heat. Add the onion, celery, carrots, and garlic, and sprinkle in the salt and oregano. Sauté the vegetables, stirring constantly until softened, about 5 minutes.

2. Add the sausage. Cook, using a spatula to crumble the sausage, until it is cooked through and browned, 5 to 8 minutes.

3. Add the bone broth, cover, and reduce the heat to medium-low. Simmer for at least 20 minutes. Stir in the kale and cook until wilted. Taste and season with more salt if needed. Enjoy warm.

4. Store any leftover soup in an airtight container in the refrigerator for up to 3 to 4 days or in the freezer for up to 3 months.

Ingredient Spotlight: Make sure to use the darker lacinato kale, which is also called dinosaur or Tuscan kale. It has the perfect taste and texture for this soup. Check the pork sausage label to ensure the ingredients are AIP-friendly. And you can always just use ground pork instead.

Per Serving: Calories: 383; Total Fat: 14g; Total Carbs: 13g; Fiber: 3g; Net Carbs: 10g; Protein: 52g

Beef Pho

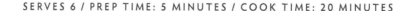

This soup is our simple AIP take on traditional Vietnamese pho. It is hot, comforting, and full of incredible flavor. We love using shirataki noodles in this recipe, which are made from glucomannan, a type of fiber from the root of the konjac plant. Swap them for zucchini noodles, if you prefer. For an extra punch of flavor, we like to garnish our soup with fresh chopped cilantro and chopped scallions.

10 cups Beef Bone Broth (store-bought or homemade, page 191)

1 (7-ounce) package shirataki noodles

1 (6-inch) piece fresh ginger, peeled and cut in half lengthwise

1 cinnamon stick

4 garlic cloves, peeled

¼ cup fish sauce

2 teaspoons raw honey

1 teaspoon pink Himalayan salt or sea salt

1 pound flank steak, finely sliced against the grain

¼ cup whole Thai basil leaves, or regular basil, torn into pieces

1 lime, cut into 6 wedges

1. In a large pot, combine the bone broth, shirataki noodles, ginger, cinnamon, garlic, fish sauce, honey, and salt. Bring the broth to a boil, then cover and reduce the heat to low. Simmer for at least 20 minutes.

2. Use a slotted spoon to remove the ginger pieces, cinnamon stick, and clove garlics from the soup, and skim off any other particles that float to the top.

3. Divide the steak, shirataki noodles, basil, cilantro, and scallions among 6 bowls and pour the hot broth into each one. The steak will cook in the broth. Serve with lime wedges.

4. Store any leftovers in an airtight container in the refrigerator for up to 3 to 4 days.

Ingredient Spotlight: Shirataki noodles can be found in the refrigerated section of the grocery store and are the perfect replacement for pasta. Plus, they contain resistant starch, which fuels your good gut bacteria. Our favorite brand is Miracle Noodles.

Per Serving: Calories: 180; Total Fat: 4g; Total Carbs: 4g; Fiber: 1g; Net Carbs: 3g; Protein: 32g

Hearty Beef Stew

SERVES 4 / PREP TIME: 5 MINUTES / COOK TIME: 35 MINUTES

We took old-fashioned beef stew and got rid of all the non-AIP thickening agents (aka flour), then upped its healing power with bone broth. This stew is a great way to use up any vegetables and fresh herbs that have been sitting around, such as zucchini, leeks, rosemary, or thyme.

1½ pounds stew beef

Pinch pink Himalayan salt or sea salt

4 tablespoons avocado oil, divided

1 cup sliced white button mushrooms

½ cup celery chopped into ½-inch pieces

½ cup yellow onion chopped into ½-inch pieces

¼ cup carrots chopped into ½-inch pieces

4 garlic cloves, minced

6 cups Beef Bone Broth (store-bought or homemade, page 191)

1 tablespoon finely chopped fresh parsley

1 teaspoon dried oregano

1 teaspoon dried thyme

1. Use paper towels to pat the stew beef dry, then season with salt.

2. In a large pot, heat 2 tablespoons of avocado oil over medium heat. Working in batches, add the beef to the pot and brown on all sides, about 4 minutes. Transfer the browned beef to a plate and set aside.

3. In the same large pot, heat the remaining 2 tablespoons of avocado oil over medium heat. Add the mushrooms, celery, onion, and carrot, and sauté for about 4 minutes, until soft. Add the garlic and sauté for an additional 1 minute.

4. Add the bone broth, parsley, oregano, thyme, and browned beef. Bring to a boil, then cover and reduce the heat to low. Simmer for 20 minutes. Enjoy immediately.

5. Store leftovers in an airtight container in the refrigerator for up to 3 to 4 days or in the freezer for up to 3 months.

Ingredient Spotlight: Stew beef is trimmed beef chuck cut into bite-size cubes; you can find it in the meat section of the supermarket. It gets more tender the longer it cooks, so the more time you let this stew simmer, the better.

Per Serving: Calories: 411; Total Fat: 21g; Total Carbs: 4g; Fiber: 1g; Net Carbs: 3g; Protein: 53g

Strawberry Bacon Spinach Salad

SERVES 1 / PREP TIME: 5 MINUTES / COOK TIME: 10 MINUTES

When fresh strawberries start showing up at the farmers' market, we know summer is officially here. We also immediately look for new and inventive ways to use them in our kitchens. This recipe came about while were experimenting with the contrast of sweet and salty flavors. The natural sweetness of the strawberries pairs perfectly with the satisfying, salty crunch of the bacon, and we can't get enough of it! Make sure to check the ingredients on the bacon package and ensure any added spices are AIP-friendly.

3 slices bacon

1 garlic clove, minced

3 cups baby spinach

½ cup strawberries, trimmed and halved

½ avocado, pitted, peeled, and diced

2 tablespoons Balsamic Vinaigrette (page 176)

1. In a large skillet, cook the bacon over medium heat for about 10 minutes, or until crisp. Transfer to a paper towel–lined plate. Coarsely chop the cooked bacon slices.

2. Put the spinach, strawberries, avocado, and bacon in a large salad bowl. Drizzle with the dressing just before serving and toss to combine. Enjoy immediately.

Make It Easier: Don't throw the bacon fat from the skillet away! Instead strain the fat into a jar and use it to make our "Cheese" Sauce (page 185) or store it in the refrigerator for up to 1 month.

Per Serving: Calories: 463; Total Fat: 34g; Total Carbs: 26g; Fiber: 12g; Net Carbs: 14g; Protein: 18g

Apple Harvest Chicken Salad

SERVES 2 / PREP TIME: 5 MINUTES / COOK TIME: 45 MINUTES

This salad is hearty, filling, and bursting with traditional fall flavors. We love making this colorful salad with crisp red apples straight from our local apple farm. The distinctly peppery flavor of arugula makes it the perfect base for this salad, but feel free to swap it out for mixed greens, spinach, or romaine if you prefer.

1 sweet potato, peeled and chopped into 1-inch cubes

2 tablespoons avocado oil

Pink Himalayan salt or sea salt

1 recipe Shredded Chicken (page 188)

4 cups arugula

2 apples, cored and diced

1 avocado, pitted, peeled, and diced

¼ red onion, diced

¼ cup Balsamic Vinaigrette (page 176)

1. Preheat the oven to 425°F. Line a large baking sheet with parchment paper.

2. Toss the sweet potato with the avocado oil and season liberally with salt. Spread in a single layer on the baking sheet, and roast in the oven for about 45 minutes, until tender.

3. Prepare the salad by tossing the roasted sweet potatoes, shredded chicken, arugula, apples, avocado, and red onion in a large bowl. Drizzle with the dressing just before serving and toss to combine. Enjoy immediately.

Make It Easier: Roast a big batch of sweet potatoes on Sunday to use throughout the week in salads or as an easy side dish. Store them in an airtight container in the refrigerator for up to 7 days. They taste great chilled in this salad, or you can reheat them if you prefer.

Per Serving: Calories: 872; Total Fat: 21g; Total Carbs: 56g; Fiber: 16g; Net Carbs: 40g; Protein: 44g

Roasted Grape Chicken Salad

SERVES 2 / PREP TIME: 5 MINUTES / COOK TIME: 20 MINUTES

If you have never tried roasted grapes, you are in for a treat! When you roast them in the oven, the grapes caramelize and develop a concentrated sweetness as they break down and release their juices. It makes them the perfect salad addition.

2 cups red seedless grapes

2 tablespoons avocado oil

¼ cup plain unsweetened coconut yogurt

1 tablespoon lemon juice

1 teaspoon dried tarragon or 1 tablespoon chopped fresh tarragon

1 teaspoon garlic powder

1 teaspoon raw honey

Pink Himalayan salt or sea salt

4 cups lacinato kale, finely chopped

1 batch Shredded Chicken (page 188)

½ cup finely sliced celery

½ cup finely sliced scallions

1. Preheat the oven to 425°F. Line a large baking sheet with parchment paper.

2. Toss the grapes with avocado oil and spread in a single layer in the pan. Roast for 15 to 20 minutes, or until they soften and burst.

3. While the grapes are roasting, make the dressing by combining the yogurt, lemon juice, tarragon, garlic powder, honey, and salt together in a medium bowl.

4. In a large salad bowl, combine the kale, chicken, celery, and scallions. Pour the dressing over everything and toss to fully mix it in. Put the bowl in the refrigerator while you wait for the grapes to finish.

5. When the grapes are done roasting, remove the salad from the refrigerator and gently fold them in. Make sure to pour the pan juices in too! This salad is best eaten right away.

Swap or Substitute: Feel free to swap out the lacinato kale for baby spinach or any mixed greens.

Per Serving: Calories: 527; Total Fat: 23g; Total Carbs: 39g; Fiber: 4g; Net Carbs: 35g; Protein: 43g

Cilantro Lime Shrimp and Avocado Salad

SERVES 1 / PREP TIME: 5 MINUTES / COOK TIME: 5 MINUTES

Cilantro is powerful detoxing herb that can accelerate the excretion of heavy metals, such as mercury and lead, from the body. As a result, we like to find new and exciting ways to get cilantro into our diet regularly. One way to do that is with this salad, which has become a regular weekday lunch for us because it can be made in just a few minutes and is absolutely delicious.

6 ounces shrimp, peeled and deveined

2 cups mixed greens

1 avocado, pitted, peeled, and diced

1 scallion, finely sliced

¼ cup Cilantro Lime Vinaigrette (page 177)

1. Fill a small pot with filtered water and bring to a boil. Add the shrimp and cook for 2 or 3 minutes, until they turn pink and become opaque. Using a strainer, drain the shrimp and immediately rinse under cold running water until they're cool to touch.

2. Put the mixed greens in a salad bowl. Top with the avocado, scallions, and cooked shrimp.

3. Drizzle the dressing onto the salad and toss to combine. Enjoy right away.

Ingredient Spotlight: You can also use precooked or frozen shrimp in this recipe. If you are using frozen shrimp, run them under cold water for 5 to 10 minutes to thaw. Then follow step 1 to cook them.

Per Serving: Calories: 629; Total Fat: 47g; Total Carbs: 31g; Fiber: 19g; Net Carbs: 12g; Protein: 32g

Salmon Niçoise Salad

Niçoise salad, with its trademark olives, is our favorite. Our version of this salad is easy to prepare, making it a great lunch or dinner option. Choose wild-caught salmon, which has the best flavor and is full of healthy fats.

2 (6-ounce) salmon fillets

Pinch pink Himalayan salt or sea salt

1 tablespoon avocado oil

2 tablespoons red wine vinegar

1 garlic clove, minced

¼ cup extra-virgin olive oil

Pinch pink Himalayan salt or sea salt

4 cups mixed greens

¼ cup peeled and diced cucumber

¼ cup thinly sliced red onion

¼ cup pitted kalamata olives

¼ cup thinly sliced red radish

1. Pat the salmon fillets dry with a paper towel, then sprinkle with salt.

2. Heat the avocado oil in a large skillet over medium heat. Add the salmon and cook for 3 to 4 minutes, carefully flip, and cook for another 3 to 4 minutes.

3. While the salmon is cooking, add the red wine vinegar and garlic into a small bowl. Stirring constantly with a fork or small whisk, slowly add the olive oil in a small, steady stream until all the oil is incorporated. Season with salt.

4. Divide the mixed greens between two salad bowls and top each with half the cucumbers, red onions, olives, radishes, and a piece of pan-seared salmon.

5. Drizzle the dressing over the salad and enjoy immediately.

Make It Easier: Feel free to use shrimp, steak, or chicken instead of salmon. Just adjust the cooking time accordingly. Or skip the cooking altogether and use canned tuna that has been drained.

Per Serving: Calories: 573; Total Fat: 44g; Total Carbs: 6g; Fiber: 2g; Net Carbs: 4g; Protein: 39g

Ginger-Marinated Seared Tuna Salad

SERVES 1 / PREP TIME: 10 MINUTES
MARINATE TIME: 10 MINUTES / COOK TIME: 6 MINUTES

Not only is this salad delicious, but it couldn't be easier to make. Unlike traditional salads, we are using cabbage and cucumber instead of lettuce as the base. Purple cabbage, also known as red cabbage, is rich in phytochemicals, vitamin C, and vitamin K. It is also high in fiber, resulting in a filling meal that's extremely satisfying.

FOR THE DRESSING

¼ cup coconut aminos

1 tablespoon avocado oil

2 teaspoons lime juice

2 garlic cloves, minced

2 teaspoons grated fresh ginger

FOR THE SALAD

1 (6-ounce) ahi tuna steak

1 tablespoon avocado oil

1 cup shredded purple cabbage

½ cucumber, peeled and diced

½ avocado, pitted, peeled, and diced

1. TO MAKE THE DRESSING: In a small bowl, combine the coconut aminos, avocado oil, lime juice, garlic, and ginger. Divide the mixture and put half in a covered container in the refrigerator.

2. Place the tuna steak in a shallow dish and pour the other half of the dressing over the top. Cover and marinate in the refrigerator for at least 10 minutes. Remove the tuna steak from the marinade and pat dry with a paper towel. Discard the marinade.

3. Heat the avocado oil in a skillet over high heat. Add the tuna steak cook for 2 to 3 minutes, carefully flip, and cook for another 2 to 3 minutes.

4. Combine the cabbage, cucumber, and avocado in a large salad bowl. Drizzle with the reserved dressing and toss to fully incorporate. Top with the cooked tuna steak and enjoy.

Ingredient Spotlight: This cooking time will result in tuna that is pink in the center. Adjust it depending on how well done you want your tuna. Look for sushi-grade ahi tuna that is fresh and high quality, especially if you prefer your tuna rare. You can also use salmon in this salad, if you prefer.

Per Serving: Calories: 713; Total Fat: 44g; Total Carbs: 28g; Fiber: 12g; Net Carbs: 16g; Protein: 55g

Greek Steak Salad

They say that the taste and smell of food can truly bring back memories. This couldn't be more true when it comes to Greek Salad. Every time we make this salad, we are immediately transported to Santorini, Greece, where we enjoyed it overlooking the crystal blue Mediterranean Sea. We use avocado in this salad rather than tomatoes to keep it AIP-friendly.

2 tablespoons avocado oil

1 (6-ounce) skirt steak

Pinch pink Himalayan salt or sea salt

2 cups mixed greens

¼ cup peeled and diced cucumber

¼ cup thinly sliced red onion

½ avocado, pitted, peeled, and diced

Juice of ½ lemon

¼ cup extra-virgin olive oil

2 teaspoons dried oregano

1. In a medium skillet, heat the avocado oil over high heat. Sprinkle the steak on both sides with salt, and then cook to your desired level of doneness: rare (2 to 3 minutes per side), medium-rare (3 to 4 minutes per side), or medium-well (5 to 7 minutes per side).

2. Transfer the steak to a cutting board and let it rest for 10 minutes.

3. As the steak rests, prepare the salad by tossing the mixed greens, cucumber, red onion, and avocado in a large bowl with the olive oil, lemon juice, and oregano. Season with salt.

4. Cut the steak, slicing against the grain, and arrange on top of the salad. Enjoy immediately.

5. Store cooked steak in an airtight container in the refrigerator for up to 3 to 4 days. Add it to the salad right before serving.

Ingredient Spotlight: Skirt steak can be a little tough, so tenderize it before cooking. Place the steak on a cutting board, cover it with plastic wrap, and use a meat tenderizer or the bottom of a heavy skillet to pound it. Don't be shy! Let it sit at room temperature for 20 minutes before cooking.

Per Serving: Calories: 1,159; Total Fat: 106g; Total Carbs: 17g; Fiber: 10g; Net Carbs: 7g; Protein: 41g

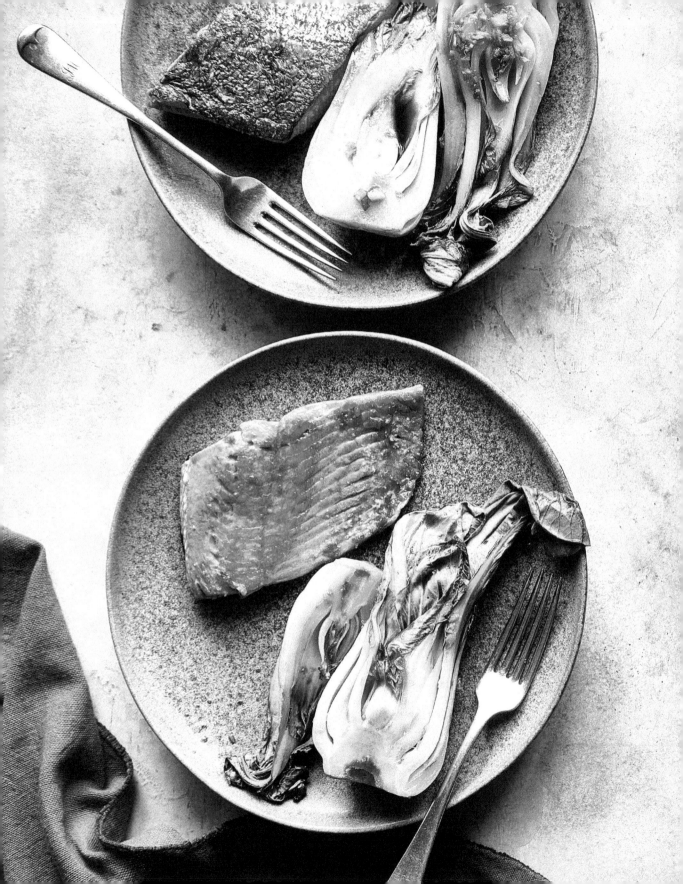

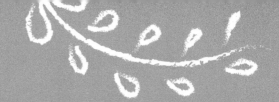

CHAPTER 6

SEAFOOD

Crispy-Skin Salmon and Ginger Bok Choy *page 112*

Turmeric-Glazed Cod and Spinach

SERVES 2 / PREP TIME: 5 MINUTES / COOK TIME: 15 MINUTES

This delicious dish cooks in one skillet, making it fast, easy, and perfect for busy weeknights. The turmeric adds a lovely earthiness without being too overpowering, and the coconut milk makes everything creamy and rich.

2 (6-ounce) cod fillets

¼ teaspoon pink Himalayan salt or sea salt

1 tablespoon coconut oil

½ small onion, thinly sliced

1 garlic clove, minced

1 cup full-fat unsweetened coconut milk (store-bought or homemade, page 174)

½ teaspoon ground turmeric

1 tablespoon coconut aminos

2 cups baby spinach

Ingredient Spotlight: The active ingredient in turmeric, curcumin, releases its powerful anti-inflammatory effects best when combined with black pepper. Black pepper is part of the AIP elimination phase, but if you have successfully reintroduced it, we suggest grinding some black pepper into the coconut milk sauce in step 2.

1. Sprinkle both sides of the cod fillets with salt.

2. In a large skillet, heat the coconut oil over medium heat. Add the onion and garlic and cook for 5 minutes, or until softened. Whisk in the coconut milk, turmeric, and coconut aminos and bring to boil. Reduce the heat and add the cod.

3. Cover and cook for 3 minutes. Then carefully flip the fish, cover, and cook for 3 to 4 more minutes, or until the internal temperature reaches 100°F.

4. Add the spinach leaves and stir. Cover again. Remove from the heat. The residual heat will cook the spinach and finish off the fish.

5. Let the pan sit, covered, until the internal temperature of the fish reaches 140° to 145°F, or when it flakes easily with a fork.

6. Serve hot. This dish is best enjoyed right away.

Per Serving: Calories: 422; Total Fat: 32g; Total Carbs: 7g; Fiber: 1g; Net Carbs: 6g; Protein: 30g

Teriyaki Sea Bass and Cauliflower Rice

SERVES 2 / PREP TIME: 5 MINUTES
MARINATE TIME: 20 MINUTES / COOK TIME: 12 MINUTES

Packed with flavor and perfect for busy weeknight dinners, this recipe has all the flavors of a traditional teriyaki but without the gluten and inflammatory ingredients. If they don't have sea bass where you buy fish, try cod or haddock.

1 garlic clove, minced

1 teaspoon grated fresh ginger

2 tablespoons coconut aminos

1 teaspoon fish sauce

2 (6-ounce) sea bass fillets

2 teaspoons coconut oil

1 cup cauliflower rice, fresh or frozen

1 scallion, thinly chopped (optional)

Make It Easier: Many grocery stores now carry premade cauliflower rice, both fresh and frozen. Thaw frozen cauliflower rice before using.

1. Whisk together the garlic, ginger, coconut aminos, and fish sauce in a shallow dish. Place the sea bass in the dish and flip to coat on both sides. Cover and place in the refrigerator to marinate for 20 minutes.

2. Heat a large skillet over medium-high heat. Add the coconut oil. Lift the fish out of the marinade and place in the skillet. Cook for 3 minutes, carefully flip, then add any remaining marinade to the skillet. Cook for 3 to 4 more minutes, until the internal temperature reaches 140° to 145°F, or when it flakes easily with a fork. Transfer the fish to a plate.

3. In the same skillet, add the cauliflower rice and sauté for about 5 minutes, or until softened.

4. Spoon the cauliflower rice alongside the sea bass and garnish with chopped scallion, if using. Serve hot.

5. Store leftovers in an airtight container in the refrigerator for up to 3 to 4 days.

Per Serving: Calories: 192; Total Fat: 7g; Total Carbs: 4g; Fiber: 1g; Net Carbs: 3g; Protein: 27g

Pesto-Crusted Halibut with Crispy Brussels Sprouts

SERVES 2 / PREP TIME: 5 MINUTES / COOK TIME: 20 MINUTES

The halibut and the Brussels sprouts in this recipe can be baked together, making this dish stress-free and easy on cleanup. To make the Brussels sprouts even more interesting, after they're cooked add some crisped bacon or pancetta, or even some pomegranate seeds, for pops of flavor and color.

2 (6-ounce) boneless, skinless halibut fillets

2 tablespoons avocado oil, divided

Pinch pink Himalayan salt or sea salt

2 tablespoons Basil-Olive Pesto (page 181), divided

½ pound Brussels sprouts, shredded

Make It Easier: Buy the Brussels sprouts pre-shredded, or shred them yourself by pulsing in a food processor.

1. Preheat the oven to 425°F. Line a large baking sheet with parchment paper.

2. Place the halibut fillets on one side of the baking sheet, rub with 1 tablespoon avocado oil, and sprinkle with salt. Evenly spread half of the pesto over the top of the fish.

3. Place the Brussels sprouts on the other side of the baking sheet and toss with the remaining 1 tablespoon oil and salt.

4. Bake for about 10 minutes, or until the internal temperature of the fish is 140°F. Transfer the fish to a plate. The fish will continue to cook, and the internal temperature should rise to 145°F. Top with the remaining pesto.

5. Continue roasting the Brussels sprouts for another 5 to 10 minutes, or until they start to crisp.

6. Plate the Brussels sprouts alongside the halibut and serve hot.

7. Store leftovers in an airtight container in the refrigerator for up to 3 to 4 days.

Per Serving: Calories: 413; Total Fat: 25g; Total Carbs: 11g; Fiber: 5g; Net Carbs: 6g; Protein: 37g

Oven-Roasted Lemon Salmon and Asparagus

SERVES 2 / PREP TIME: 5 MINUTES / COOK TIME: 15 MINUTES

This dish is one of our favorite recipes to make in the spring, when asparagus is at its best and sweetest. We love how the lemon complements the salmon and the asparagus. Perhaps the best part of this dish? Everything bakes in the same pan, so there's very little cleanup.

2 tablespoons avocado oil, divided

2 garlic cloves, minced

2 (6-ounce) salmon fillets

Juice of ½ lemon

Pinch pink Himalayan salt or sea salt

½ pound asparagus, ends trimmed

½ lemon, cut into slices

Ingredient Spotlight: Asparagus contains high levels of asparagine, an amino acid that is a natural diuretic. Asparagine can help flush the body of excess fluid, helping to relieve bloating, and can aid in preventing urinary tract infections.

1. Preheat the oven to 425°F. Line a baking sheet with parchment paper.

2. In a small bowl, combine 1 tablespoon of the avocado oil and the minced garlic.

3. Place the salmon fillets on the baking sheet and rub with the garlic and oil mixture to evenly coat. Squeeze the lemon juice over the salmon and season with salt.

4. Arrange the asparagus around the salmon in a single layer. Drizzle the spears with the remaining 1 tablespoon of avocado oil, and cover with the lemon slices.

5. Roast for 12 to 15 minutes, until the salmon is cooked through to your liking and you can easily flake the fish with a fork. Serve hot.

6. Store leftovers in an airtight container in the refrigerator for up to 3 to 4 days.

Per Serving: Calories: 395; Total Fat: 25g; Total Carbs: 6g; Fiber: 3g; Net Carbs: 3g; Protein: 36g

Crispy-Skin Salmon and Ginger Bok Choy

SERVES 2 / PREP TIME: 7 MINUTES
MARINATE TIME: 20 MINUTES / COOK TIME: 10 MINUTES

Perfectly crisped salmon skin is the star of this healthy and delicious dish. We love the sweetness from the coconut aminos and the fresh and zesty flavors of the ginger. Pair it with tender baby bok choy for a complete and healthy meal.

½ pound salmon fillet, skin on

¼ teaspoon pink Himalayan salt or sea salt

1 teaspoon grated fresh ginger

2 tablespoons coconut aminos, plus 2 teaspoons

3 teaspoons coconut oil, divided

3 garlic cloves, minced

1 teaspoon minced fresh ginger

½ pound baby bok choy, cut in half lengthwise

1. Pat the salmon skin dry with a paper towel and sprinkle with salt.

2. In a large, shallow dish, whisk together the ginger and coconut aminos. Place the salmon flesh-side down in the mixture, cover, and marinate in the refrigerator for 20 minutes.

3. While the salmon marinates, start on the bok choy. Heat a large skillet over medium-high heat and pour in 2 teaspoons of coconut oil. Add the garlic and ginger, and sauté for 1 to 2 minutes. Then add the bok choy and coconut aminos. Toss the bok choy to coat it in the sauce, cook for another 1 to 2 minutes, or until slightly wilted. Transfer the bok choy to a bowl and tent it with aluminum foil to keep warm while you cook the salmon.

4. In the same skillet, add the remaining 1 teaspoon of coconut oil and turn the heat to medium. Place the salmon skin-side down in the skillet and cook for about 6 minutes, or until it is mostly cooked through. Reduce the heat if it appears the salmon skin is blackening.

5. Flip the salmon and pour the marinade in the bottom of the pan, making sure not to let the marinade touch the crispy skin. Reduce the heat to low and cook for 1 or 2 more minutes, until the internal temperature reaches 140°F (the temperature should continue to rise to 145°F) or when it flakes easily with a fork.

6. Cut the salmon in half and transfer to a serving plate. Serve hot alongside the bok choy.

7. Store leftovers in an airtight container in the refrigerator for up to 3 to 4 days.

Ingredient Spotlight: The skin of the salmon contains the highest concentration of inflammation-fighting omega-3 fatty acids.

Per Serving: Calories: 250; Total Fat: 14g; Total Carbs: 5g; Fiber: 1g; Net Carbs: 4g; Protein: 26g

Salmon Burgers with Sweet Potato Oven Fries

SERVES 4 / PREP TIME: 15 MINUTES
SOAK TIME: 30 MINUTES / COOK TIME: 30 MINUTES

This AIP-friendly recipe is perfect for when you have those cravings for a fast-food burger and fries. Made with all anti-inflammatory ingredients, this dish makes for a delicious and healthy lunch or dinner. Make the burgers in a skillet indoors, or use a grill if you are having an outdoor cookout. And, of course, you can make the oven fries any time, including on their own as a snack.

FOR THE SWEET POTATO OVEN FRIES

2 large sweet potatoes, peeled and cut into thin strips

2 tablespoons arrowroot starch

3 tablespoons avocado oil

1 teaspoon pink Himalayan salt or sea salt

¼ teaspoon garlic powder

TO MAKE THE SWEET POTATO OVEN FRIES

1. Put the sweet potato strips in a bowl of cold filtered water and let sit for 30 minutes. Drain and pat dry with paper towels.

2. Preheat the oven to 400°F. Line two large baking sheets with parchment paper

3. Put the sweet potato strips in a large bowl and toss with arrowroot starch until they are evenly coated. Spread them out on the baking sheets and toss gently with the oil, salt, and garlic powder. Space the strips apart so that they are not touching one another. Bake for 30 minutes, or until slightly browned and crispy.

1½ pounds boneless, skinless salmon

1 shallot, roughly chopped

1 tablespoon capers, drained

2 tablespoons coconut aminos

½ teaspoon pink Himalayan salt or sea salt

1 tablespoon avocado oil

2 cups mixed greens

¼ cup Classic Ranch Dressing (page 178)

2 tablespoons chopped dill (optional)

4. While the sweet potato fries are baking, prepare the burgers. Put one-quarter of the salmon in a food processor or blender, along with the shallot, capers, coconut aminos, and salt. Pulse until it becomes a paste but before it turns to liquid. Add the remaining salmon and pulse until the fish is well chopped and combined with the paste. Form into 4 patties.

5. Heat the avocado oil a large skillet over medium-high heat. Then add the salmon burgers and cook for about 3 minutes on each side, checking to make sure they are mostly cooked through but still pink in the center.

6. To serve, divide the mixed greens among four plates and place the burgers on top of the greens. Spoon 1 tablespoon of ranch dressing on top of each burger. Garnish with chopped dill, if using. Serve with the sweet potato fries.

7. Store leftovers in a sealed container in the refrigerator for up to 3 to 4 days.

Make It Easier: To save on time, replace the fresh salmon with 2 (14-ounce) cans of salmon. Then you can skip the food processor and just mash it all with a fork in a big bowl.

Per Serving: Calories: 468; Total Fat: 27g; Total Carbs: 18g; Fiber: 3g; Net Carbs: 15g; Protein: 36g

Sushi-Style Tuna Steaks with Cucumber Avocado Salad

SERVES 2 / PREP TIME: 10 MINUTES
MARINATE TIME: 25 MINUTES / COOK TIME: 5 MINUTES

People on an anti-inflammatory diet often miss spicy foods, but this dish will give you that spicy fix you've been craving, courtesy of wasabi. If you have reintroduced seeds, crust the tuna steaks with 6 tablespoons of black and white sesame seeds after marinating and before searing. Make the vinaigrette and mayo ahead of time so the dish comes together quickly and with minimal effort.

FOR THE TUNA

2 garlic cloves, minced

2 teaspoons grated fresh ginger

2 tablespoons coconut aminos

2 teaspoons fish sauce

1 tablespoon coconut oil

2 (6-ounce) tuna steaks

3 tablespoons AIP Mayo (page 179)

2 teaspoons wasabi paste

FOR THE CUCUMBER AVOCADO SALAD

1 avocado, pitted, peeled, and diced

1 cucumber, chopped

½ cucumber, diced

2 tablespoons Cilantro Lime Vinaigrette (page 177)

1. In a large shallow dish, whisk together the garlic, ginger, coconut aminos, and fish sauce. Place the tuna steaks in the marinade and flip them to coat both sides. Cover the dish and marinate in the refrigerator for 25 minutes.

2. **TO MAKE THE CUCUMBER AVOCADO SALAD:** In a large bowl, lightly toss the avocado, cucumber, and vinaigrette. Refrigerate.

3. Heat the coconut oil in a large skillet over high heat. Sear the tuna steaks for about 2 minutes on each side, making sure to keep the insides pink and rare.

4. Arrange the chilled salad alongside the tuna steaks on two dinner plates. Combine the mayo and wasabi paste in a small bowl for dipping.

Ingredient Spotlight: Always check to make sure the wasabi paste is made with all AIP-friendly ingredients. Try using the powder form if you can't find the paste. Wasabi powder is readily available in most grocery stores and can be formed into a paste by mixing it with a bit of filtered water.

Per Serving: Calories: 649; Total Fat: 44g; Total Carbs: 19g; Fiber: 10g; Net Carbs: 9g; Protein: 48g

Shrimp Fried Rice

SERVES 4 / PREP TIME: 10 MINUTES / COOK TIME: 10 MINUTES

We sometimes call this Fried-ay Rice because we usually make this on Friday nights when we are trying to use up any extra veggies in the refrigerator. This is a recipe your whole family will love, and a great way to get your kids to eat their vegetables. You won't be missing the takeout version when you make this delicious dish. Make a large batch and enjoy it as leftovers the next day.

1 tablespoon coconut oil

2 garlic cloves, minced

1 medium onion, diced

½ cup diced zucchini

½ cup chopped mushrooms

½ cup diced carrots

6 cups cauliflower rice

1 pound medium shrimp, peeled and deveined

¼ cup coconut aminos

1 tablespoon fish sauce

Pinch pink Himalayan salt or sea salt

2 scallions, chopped, for garnishing (optional)

1. Heat the coconut oil in a large skillet over medium heat. Stir in the garlic, onion, zucchini, mushrooms, and carrots. Cook for 5 minutes, then add the cauliflower rice. Cook for another 3 minutes. Add the shrimp and cook for 2 minutes.

2. Stir in the coconut aminos and fish sauce and cook for another 2 or 3 minutes, stirring frequently to coat the vegetables and shrimp in the sauce. Add a pinch of salt, if needed.

3. Serve hot, garnished with scallions, if using.

4. Store the leftovers in an airtight container in the refrigerator for up to 3 to 4 days.

Swap or Substitute: This dish is so versatile, you can add many different vegetables and proteins. Try replacing the shrimp with cooked chicken or pork. You can also add some broccoli florets or shallots. If you have reintroduced eggs, move the vegetables and shrimp to one side of the skillet and lightly scramble 2 eggs. Stir it all together when the eggs have cooked.

Per Serving: Calories: 186; Total Fat: 5g; Total Carbs: 15g; Fiber: 5g; Net Carbs: 10g; Protein: 22g

Shrimp Scampi with Zucchini Noodles

SERVES 2 / PREP TIME: 5 MINUTES
MARINATE TIME: 20 MINUTES / COOK TIME: 15 MINUTES

This dish is elegant enough to serve at a dinner party, but also easy enough to make as a quick and comforting weeknight meal. Any size shrimp will work with this recipe, from small all the way to jumbo. Switch out the avocado oil for butter or ghee if you have successfully reintroduced dairy. Another great garnish option if you have reintroduced dairy is shredded or grated Parmesan cheese.

2 tablespoons avocado oil

2 tablespoons lemon juice

2 tablespoons coconut aminos

2 garlic cloves, minced

¼ teaspoon dried oregano

2 tablespoons chopped fresh parsley (optional)

½ pound shrimp, peeled and deveined

1 zucchini, spiralized or cut into noodles and dried with paper towels

Make It Easier: Most grocery stores sell spiralized zucchini noodles fresh in the produce section and frozen in the freezer aisle.

1. In a large shallow dish, whisk together the oil, lemon juice, coconut aminos, garlic, oregano, and parsley (if using). Add the shrimp and toss to coat. Cover and marinate in the refrigerator for 20 minutes.

2. Meanwhile, preheat the oven to 250°F and line a large baking sheet with parchment paper.

3. Spread out the zucchini noodles on the baking sheet and bake them for 10 minutes to help remove some of the moisture. Remove them from the oven and set aside.

4. Heat a large skillet over medium heat. Add the shrimp and the marinade. Cook for about 5 minutes, or until the shrimp are cooked through. Gently mix the zucchini noodles into the shrimp and toss to coat with the sauce.

5. Serve hot.

6. Store leftovers in an airtight container in the refrigerator for up to 3 to 4 days.

Per Serving: Calories: 240; Total Fat: 16g; Total Carbs: 7g; Fiber: 1g; Net Carbs: 6g; Protein: 19g

Lime Shrimp Kebabs over Mixed Greens

SERVES 2 / PREP TIME: 10 MINUTES
MARINATE TIME: 25 MINUTES / COOK TIME: 5 MINUTES

For a fresh lunch or dinner dish, you'll love these zesty kebabs. Grill them on an outdoor grill on a sunny day, or cook them under a broiler if you don't have a grill or you just don't feel like cooking outside. Add sliced avocado, shredded carrots, or thinly sliced radishes for a more complete salad with beautiful pops of color.

1 tablespoon avocado oil

2 tablespoons lime juice

1 tablespoon coconut aminos

1 garlic clove, minced

⅛ teaspoon pink Himalayan salt or sea salt

½ pound shrimp, peeled and deveined

3 cups mixed greens

2 tablespoons Cilantro Lime Vinaigrette (page 177)

Swap or Substitute: Substitute Classic Ranch Dressing (page 178) for Cilantro Lime Vinaigrette and swap out the lime juice for lemon for a different take on this dish.

1. In a shallow glass dish, whisk together the oil, lime juice, coconut aminos, garlic, and salt. Add the shrimp and toss to coat. Cover and marinate in the refrigerator for 25 minutes.

2. Preheat the grill to medium heat, or set a rack 4 inches from the broiling element and preheat the broiler.

3. Skewer the shrimp on 6 metal skewers or 6 wooden skewers that have been soaked in water for at least 10 minutes. Discard the marinade.

4. Grill the kebabs, covered, for about 4 minutes. Or place the kebabs on a sheet pan and broil in the oven for 5 to 6 minutes.

5. Divide the mixed greens evenly among 2 shallow bowls and drizzle with the vinaigrette. Top each salad with 3 kebabs. Serve while the shrimp is hot.

6. Store leftovers in an airtight container in the refrigerator for up to 3 to 4 days.

Per Serving: Calories: 224; Total Fat: 15g; Total Carbs: 6g; Fiber: 1g; Net Carbs: 5g; Protein: 18g

Grilled Chimichurri Shrimp and Cucumber Mint Salad

SERVES 4 / PREP TIME: 5 MINUTES
MARINATE TIME: 45 MINUTES / COOK TIME: 5 MINUTES

This dish is full of fresh flavors and is perfect for grilling at an outdoor barbecue. Double the recipe if you are serving a larger crowd. We love serving this dish at summer cookouts. The cool cucumbers and mint are so refreshing on hot and humid evenings.

2 tablespoons avocado oil

1 tablespoon coconut aminos

4 tablespoons Chimichurri (page 182), divided

½ pound jumbo shrimp, peeled and deveined

1 cucumber, chopped

1 radish, thinly sliced

½ cup chopped fresh mint leaves

2 tablespoons Cilantro Lime Vinaigrette (page 177)

Ingredient Spotlight: Cilantro is packed with calcium, potassium, magnesium, folate, and vitamins A, C, and K. It has many anti-inflammatory properties and can even bind to heavy metals and remove them from the body.

1. In a large shallow glass dish, whisk together the avocado oil, coconut aminos, and 2 tablespoons of the chimichurri. Place the shrimp in the marinade and flip to coat on both sides. Cover and marinate in the refrigerator for 45 minutes.

2. While the shrimp marinates, prepare the cucumber mint salad. Toss the cucumber, radish, mint, and vinaigrette together in a large bowl. Refrigerate.

3. Heat the grill to medium-high heat, or heat a large cast iron skillet on the stovetop over medium-high heat.

4. Cook the shrimp on the grill or skillet for about 3 minutes on each side. Remove from the heat and pour the remaining 2 tablespoons of chimichurri over the shrimp. Serve alongside the cucumber mint salad.

5. Store leftovers in an airtight container in the refrigerator for up to 3 to 4 days.

Per Serving: Calories: 237; Total Fat: 21g; Total Carbs: 3g; Fiber: 0g; Net Carbs: 3g; Protein: 9g

Steamed Mussels with Garlic Dipping Bread

SERVES 2 / PREP TIME: 5 MINUTES / COOK TIME: 35 MINUTES

Mussels have anti-inflammatory properties that can help prevent asthma and reduce arthritis. The omega-3 fatty acids, DHA, and B₁₂ found in mussels can improve brain health and memory as you age. Remember to discard the mussels that have already opened before you start cooking, as this indicates they are not safe to eat.

2 teaspoons coconut oil

1 shallot, thinly sliced

2 garlic cloves, minced

2 teaspoons grated fresh ginger

2 teaspoons white wine vinegar

2⅔ cups full-fat unsweetened coconut milk (store-bought or homemade, page 174)

2 tablespoons coconut aminos

1 tablespoon fish sauce

Pinch pink Himalayan salt or sea salt

2 pounds live mussels, cleaned

¼ cup chopped fresh cilantro (optional)

1 scallion, diced (optional)

2 AIP Garlic Herb Flatbreads (page 62), sliced lengthwise into breadsticks

1. In a large pot, melt the coconut oil on medium heat. Add the shallot, garlic, and ginger and cook for 3 to 5 minutes, or until softened. Then stir in the vinegar and cook for another 2 or 3 minutes.

2. Stir in the coconut milk, coconut aminos, and fish sauce. Season with salt. Increase the heat to medium-high.

3. Add the mussels and cover the pot. Cook for 5 to 7 minutes, or until the mussels have opened. Some may take more time to open or may not open at all. Discard those that don't open.

4. Transfer the mussels to a large, shallow bowl, stir in the cilantro, and garnish with scallion, if using. Serve with the flatbread sticks on the side to dip into the sauce.

Swap or Substitute: For some heat in the sauce, add a couple of teaspoons of hot sauce or 1 tablespoon of curry paste in step 2, if you have successfully reintroduced nightshades and spices.

Per Serving: Calories: 1,000; Total Fat: 89g; Total Carbs: 36g; Fiber: 1g; Net Carbs: 35g; Protein: 25g

Pan-Seared Scallops and Roasted Garlic Broccoli

SERVES 2 / PREP TIME: 5 MINUTES / COOK TIME: 20 MINUTES

The tastiest way to cook scallops is to pan sear them in a little oil. The outsides get a nice crisp and they develop a lovely sweet flavor. And the best part? They cook so quickly. We love this dish for its elegance and simplicity—and because there is hardly any cleanup.

½ pound broccoli florets

2 tablespoons coconut oil

2 garlic cloves, minced

1 teaspoon pink Himalayan salt or sea salt

½ pound sea scallops, patted dry

½ teaspoon pink Himalayan salt or sea salt

2 teaspoons avocado oil

1. Preheat the oven to 400°F.

2. Put the broccoli on a large sheet pan and toss with the coconut oil, garlic, and salt. Bake for 20 minutes, or until the broccoli is starting to brown on the tops.

3. When the broccoli has cooked for 10 minutes, start cooking the scallops. Sprinkle both sides of the scallops with salt.

4. Heat a large skillet over high heat and pour in the avocado oil. When the oil is shimmering, place the scallops in a single layer in the skillet. Cook on each side for 2 to 3 minutes, or until browned.

5. Remove and serve with the roasted broccoli.

6. Store leftovers in an airtight container in the refrigerator for up to 3 to 4 days.

Ingredient Spotlight: The vitamin B_{12} in scallops can lower homocysteine levels in the blood, which can reduce inflammation in the blood vessels and help prevent heart attacks and strokes.

Per Serving: Calories: 280; Total Fat: 19g; Total Carbs: 12g; Fiber: 3g; Net Carbs: 9g; Protein: 17g

Crab-Stuffed Mushrooms and Roasted Asparagus

SERVES 2 / PREP TIME: 10 MINUTES / COOK TIME: 20 MINUTES

Serve this elegant dish for a special dinner date at home or for a dinner party when you're feeling up to hosting. Try to find fresh lump or jumbo lump crabmeat and avoid the crabmeat that is sold in cans. We prefer blue crabmeat in this recipe for its sweet flavor and tender lumps of meat.

4 ounces lump or jumbo lump crabmeat

2 tablespoons AIP Mayo (page 179)

⅛ teaspoon garlic powder

2 large portobello mushrooms, stems and gills removed and tops wiped clean

2 teaspoons avocado oil, plus 1 tablespoon

Pinch pink Himalayan salt or sea salt

½ pound asparagus, ends trimmed

Ingredient Spotlight: Crabs are a crustacean that contain high levels of phosphorus, which can help improve kidney function. This can help promote the release of toxins in the body, making them a great seafood choice for people with autoimmune disease.

1. Preheat the oven to 375°F.

2. In a medium bowl, carefully mix together the crabmeat, mayo, and garlic powder, being careful not to break apart the crab lumps.

3. Place the mushrooms on one side of a large baking sheet and rub each one with 1 teaspoon of avocado oil. Sprinkle with salt. Spoon the crab mixture evenly into the mushroom caps. On the same baking dish, toss together the asparagus, the remaining 1 tablespoon of avocado oil, and salt.

4. Bake for about 20 minutes, or until the tops of the asparagus have crisped slightly and the crab mixture is heated through.

5. Remove the mushrooms and asparagus from oven and serve together.

6. Store leftovers in an airtight container in the refrigerator for up to 3 to 4 days.

Per Serving: Calories: 340; Total Fat: 27g; Total Carbs: 11g; Fiber: 5g; Net Carbs: 6g; Protein: 19g

Creamy Lobster Pasta over Shirataki Noodles

SERVES 2 TO 3 / PREP TIME: 10 MINUTES / COOK TIME: 40 MINUTES

This hearty and filling pasta dish is sure to appeal to everyone—even kids! Shirataki noodles make a wonderful replacement to traditional noodles made with grains. They cook quickly and can take on the flavors of a sauce nicely. Use either angel hair or fettuccine shirataki noodles for this recipe. To keep costs low, feel free to swap the lobster in this recipe with cooked shrimp.

2 (7-ounce) packages angel hair or fettuccine shirataki noodles

1 tablespoon avocado oil

2 shallots, diced

2 garlic cloves, minced

¼ cup chopped celery

¼ cup chopped carrots

1 bay leaf

2 teaspoons apple cider vinegar

1½ cups Chicken Bone Broth (store-bought or homemade, page 190)

1 cup coconut cream

1 pound cooked lobster meat

1. Prepare the shirataki noodles according to the package instructions. Set aside

2. Heat a large pot over medium heat and pour in the oil. Stir in the shallots, garlic, celery, carrot, and bay leaf. Sauté for 5 minutes, or until softened. Stir in the vinegar and cook for another 3 minutes.

3. Add the broth and coconut cream. Turn the heat up to medium-high and bring to a boil, then reduce the heat and simmer for 20 minutes so the sauce can thicken.

4. Stir in the lobster meat and cooked noodles and cook on low for 10 minutes. Serve hot.

5. Store leftovers in an airtight container in the refrigerator for up to 3 to 4 days.

Ingredient Spotlight: Shirataki noodles are a popular replacement for pasta for people who are following an AIP or a low-carb diet. They are made from the konjac root and are a natural source of fiber, which can aid in digestive health. You can find shirataki noodles at some grocery stores or you can buy them online. If you cannot find shirataki noodles, use spaghetti squash or zucchini noodles.

Per Serving: Calories: 680; Total Fat: 51g; Total Carbs: 12g; Fiber: 4g; Net Carbs: 8g; Protein: 48g

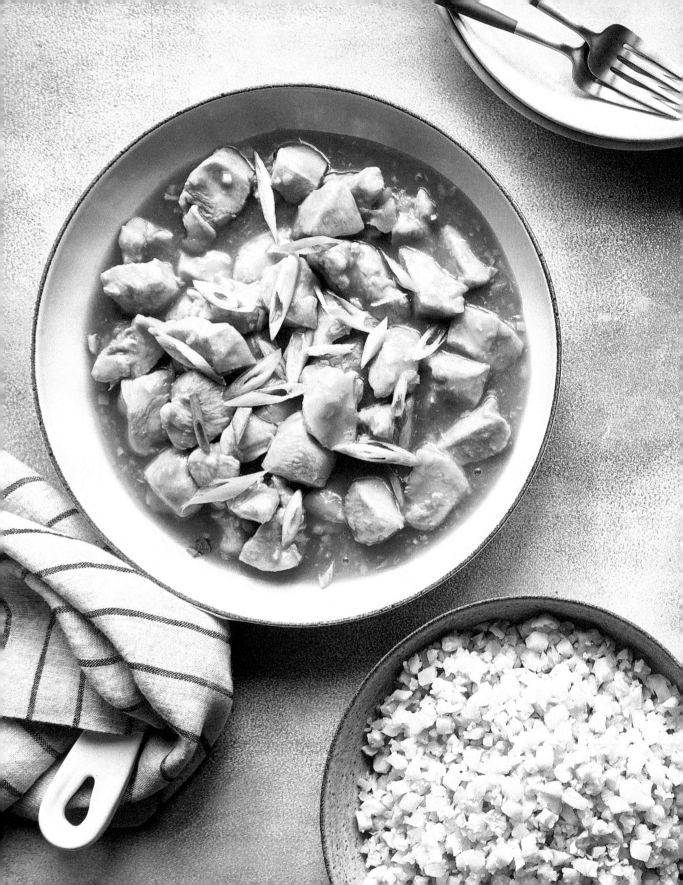

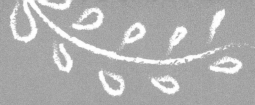

CHAPTER 7

POULTRY

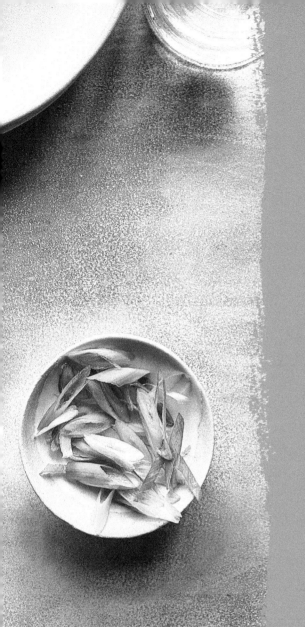

Orange Chicken with Cauliflower Rice *page 132*

Chicken and Vegetables Sheet Pan Supper

SERVES 4 / PREP TIME: 5 MINUTES
MARINATE TIME: 20 MINUTES / COOK TIME: 20 MINUTES

This recipe cooks on one sheet pan and is perfect for busy weeknights when you don't feel like fussing. And the best part? Minimal cleanup! Make a large batch to eat as leftovers throughout the week, or freeze the extras and enjoy them later when you want a hearty dinner in a hurry.

¼ cup coconut aminos

2 tablespoons raw honey

3 garlic cloves, minced, divided

2 tablespoons avocado oil, divided

1 pound boneless, skinless chicken breasts, cut into 1-inch pieces

1 large head broccoli, cut into florets

2 large carrots, cut into 1-inch pieces

1 teaspoon pink Himalayan salt or sea salt

¼ cup Classic Ranch Dressing (page 178)

1. In a small bowl, whisk together the coconut aminos, honey, 2 cloves of minced garlic, and 1 tablespoon of the oil. Transfer to a shallow dish and add the chicken. Toss to coat. Cover the dish and marinate in the refrigerator for at least 20 minutes.

2. Preheat the oven to 375°F.

3. On a large sheet pan, toss together the broccoli, carrots, salt, remaining 1 clove of minced garlic, and remaining 1 tablespoon of oil. Transfer the chicken to the sheet pan and mix with the vegetables, reserving the marinade. Bake for about 20 minutes, or until the internal temperature of the chicken reaches 165°F.

4. While the chicken is baking, put the marinade in a small saucepan over medium-low heat. Let it bubble and thicken for 5 to 10 minutes.

5. Remove the sheet pan from the oven, pour the sauce over the chicken and vegetables, and toss to combine.

6. Drizzle with the ranch dressing over everything and serve hot.

7. Store leftovers in an airtight container in the refrigerator for up to 3 to 4 days or in the freezer for up to 3 months.

Swap or Substitute: If you're looking to mix things up, replace the broccoli and carrots with zucchini, cauliflower, or mushrooms.

Per Serving: Calories: 304; Total Fat: 10g; Total Carbs: 24g; Fiber: 5g; Net Carbs: 19g; Protein: 33g

"Cheesy" Chicken and Broccoli Casserole

SERVES 4 / PREP TIME: 10 MINUTES / COOK TIME: 33 MINUTES

Prepackaged cauliflower rice is available in most grocery stores. We love having it ready to use in a variety of recipes. If you can't find it, grate a head of cauliflower with a box grater to make the cauliflower rice, or chop a head of cauliflower into florets and add them to a food processor and pulse until you have rice-size pieces.

2 teaspoons avocado oil

1 small onion, diced

2 garlic cloves, minced

4 cups broccoli florets

1 pound boneless, skinless chicken breasts, cut into 1-inch pieces

2 cups cauliflower rice

1½ cups "Cheese" Sauce (page 185)

1. Preheat the oven to 350°F.

2. In a large skillet over medium heat, combine the avocado oil, onion, and garlic. Cook for 4 to 5 minutes, or until softened. Add the broccoli and cook for another 4 to 5 minutes. Add the chicken and cook until the chicken is almost cooked through, about 5 minutes. Stir in the cauliflower rice and cook for 2 or 3 more minutes.

3. Add the "Cheese" Sauce and mix until the chicken and vegetables are coated.

4. Transfer the mixture to a 9-by-11-inch casserole dish and bake for 15 minutes. Serve hot.

5. Store leftovers in an airtight container in the refrigerator for up to 3 to 4 days or in the freezer for up to 3 months.

Make It Easier: To make this dish even easier, skip the baking and just enjoy it hot right after you mix in the "Cheese" Sauce in step 3.

Per Serving: Calories: 305; Total Fat: 14g; Total Carbs: 16g; Fiber: 9g; Net Carbs: 7g; Protein: 32g

Creamy Chicken and "Rice" Casserole

SERVES 4 / PREP TIME: 5 MINUTES / COOK TIME: 20 MINUTES

This hearty and warming dish is sure to become a family favorite. It's like a cross between chicken soup and chicken pot pie, and the result is a delicious recipe that you will come back to time and time again. You'll love how much the shirataki rice actually tastes like the real thing.

2 (7-ounce) packages shirataki rice

½ cup lard

⅓ cup cassava flour

1 garlic clove, minced

½ cup diced onion

½ cup diced carrots

½ cup diced celery

½ teaspoon dried thyme or 2 teaspoons chopped fresh thyme

1 teaspoon pink Himalayan salt or sea salt

1½ cups chicken broth or chicken bone broth (store-bought or homemade, page 190)

1 pound chicken breasts, cooked and shredded, or Shredded Chicken (page 188)

1. Prepare the shirataki rice according to the package instructions. Set aside.

2. Heat a large skillet over medium-low heat and melt the lard. When it's melted, stir in the cassava flour and cook for 3 to 5 minutes, stirring constantly and making sure the flour isn't turning dark brown.

3. Add the garlic, onion, carrot, and celery and cook until softened, about 5 minutes. Stir in the thyme, salt, broth, chicken, and rice. Turn the heat up to medium and simmer for 10 minutes. Serve hot.

4. Store leftovers in an airtight container in the refrigerator for up to 3 to 4 days or in the freezer for up to 3 months.

Swap or Substitute: Replace the lard with equal amounts of butter, if you have been able to successfully reintroduce it into your diet. The chicken breasts can be replaced with the same amount of boneless, skinless chicken thighs. The shirataki rice can easily be swapped for 3 cups of cauliflower rice.

Per Serving: Calories: 442; Total Fat: 29g; Total Carbs: 14g; Fiber: 2g; Net Carbs: 12g; Protein: 32g

Orange Chicken with Cauliflower Rice

Our anti-inflammatory spin on the Chinese takeout classic is every bit as delicious. Even better is that the house will smell fabulous from all the fresh orange zest and ginger. This is another dish where you can substitute two (14-ounce) packages of shirataki rice for the cauliflower rice and have equally fabulous results.

½ cup arrowroot starch

4 boneless, skinless chicken breasts, cut into 1-inch pieces

2 teaspoons coconut oil

2 garlic cloves, minced

1 teaspoon grated fresh ginger

Zest of 1 orange

1 cup orange juice

¼ cup raw honey

2 tablespoons white wine vinegar

2 tablespoons coconut aminos

2 cups cauliflower rice

2 scallions, chopped (optional)

1. Place the arrowroot starch in a medium bowl and dredge chicken pieces in it to fully coat. Set aside.

2. In a large skillet over medium heat, heat the coconut oil. Stir in the garlic and ginger and cook for 3 minutes. Stir in the orange zest, orange juice, honey, vinegar, and coconut aminos. Bring the sauce to a simmer and cook for 10 minutes.

3. Add the chicken and stir to coat in the sauce. Cook for 15 minutes, or until the chicken is cooked through.

4. While the chicken is cooking, prepare the cauliflower rice by placing a steamer basket inside a large pot filled with just enough filtered water to touch the bottom of the basket. Add the cauliflower rice to the basket and cover. Bring the water to a boil and cook for 5 minutes, or until the rice is softened.

5. Divide the cauliflower rice among four plates or bowls. Top with the chicken and sauce, then garnish with chopped scallions, if using.

6. Store leftovers in an airtight container in the refrigerator for up to 3 to 4 days or in the freezer for up to 3 months.

Ingredient Spotlight: The beta-carotene in oranges prevents free radicals from damaging your skin. The inflammation that occurs with autoimmune disease can affect the skin, so foods high in antioxidants, such as oranges, are an important part of an anti-inflammatory diet.

Per Serving: Calories: 274; Total Fat: 4g; Total Carbs: 30g; Fiber: 2g; Net Carbs: 28g; Protein: 30g

Crispy-Skin Chicken Thighs with Coleslaw

SERVES 4 / PREP TIME: 5 MINUTES / COOK TIME: 40 MINUTES

Crispy chicken skin is the star of this easy and delicious meal. We love the slightly sweet sauce that's drizzled over the chicken and the cool, refreshing coleslaw that completes this meal. These chicken thighs are baked in the oven, so you don't have to do much in the kitchen. If you're not in the mood for coleslaw, serve the chicken with any easy side dish or a simple salad. And this slaw is great with many different dishes, including Oven-Fried Chicken Nuggets (page 64) and Sticky Orange Wings (page 65).

FOR THE CHICKEN

8 skin-on, bone-in chicken thighs

2 tablespoons avocado oil

3 teaspoons pink Himalayan salt or sea salt, divided

3 tablespoons coconut aminos

2 tablespoons raw honey

1 tablespoon white wine vinegar

½ cup apple cider vinegar

FOR THE COLESLAW

2 tablespoons coconut sugar

2 tablespoons extra-virgin olive oil

1 (14-ounce) bag coleslaw mix

1. Preheat the oven to 425°F. Place a metal rack on top of a foil-lined baking sheet to prevent the thighs from sitting in their own grease as they cook.

2. Pat the chicken dry with paper towels, rub them all over with the avocado oil, and sprinkle evenly with 2 teaspoons salt. Lay the chicken on the rack.

3. Bake for 35 to 40 minutes, or until the internal temperature reaches 165°F to 170°F and the skin is crispy and golden brown.

4. While the chicken bakes, prepare the sauce by combining the coconut aminos, honey, and white wine vinegar in a small saucepan over medium-low heat. Bring the mixture to a simmer, then reduce the heat to low and simmer for 10 minutes to thicken the sauce. Set aside.

5. TO MAKE THE COLESLAW: In a large bowl, whisk together the apple cider vinegar, coconut sugar, olive oil, and remaining 1 teaspoon of salt. Pour the bag of coleslaw mix into the bowl, and toss to combine. Refrigerate until the chicken finishes cooking.

6. If the chicken skin is not crisping, try sticking the thighs under the broiler for 3 to 4 minutes to help them develop a crunch. Drizzle the sauce over the thighs and serve alongside the coleslaw.

7. Store leftover thighs and coleslaw in separate airtight containers in the refrigerator for up to 3 to 4 days or in the freezer for up to 3 months.

Swap or Substitute: You can swap out the shredded cabbage mix for shredded broccoli mix. Also, if packaged bags aren't available, you can shred the cabbage by quickly pulsing it in a food processor.

Per Serving: Calories: 720; Total Fat: 51g; Total Carbs: 22g; Fiber: 3g; Net Carbs: 19g; Protein: 40g

Chicken Fingers with Rosemary Honey over Mixed Greens

SERVES 4 / PREP TIME: 10 MINUTES / COOK TIME: 20 MINUTES

These chicken fingers are baked instead of fried, which makes them easy to make and easy to clean up. To shorten the prep time, use bags of crushed pork rinds. If you can't find them, crush the pork rinds in a food processor or with your hands.

1½ cups crushed pork rinds

½ cup cassava flour

¼ cup arrowroot starch

1 teaspoon garlic powder

1 teaspoon onion powder

1½ pounds chicken tenders, cut in half lengthwise

3 tablespoons raw honey

2 tablespoons coconut aminos

½ teaspoon dried rosemary or 2 teaspoons chopped fresh rosemary

6 cups mixed greens

Ingredient Spotlight: The antioxidant compounds in honey have been linked to lower blood pressure and an improvement in cholesterol levels. Honey is a great substitute for refined sugar as it does not raise blood sugar levels as much.

1. Preheat the oven to 375°F. Line a baking sheet with parchment paper and set aside.

2. In a shallow dish, mix together pork rinds, cassava flour, arrowroot starch, garlic powder, and onion powder. Dredge the chicken in the mixture and set on the baking sheet, making sure the pieces are separated.

3. Bake for 20 to 25 minutes, or until crisped and golden brown and the internal temperature is 160°F to 165°F.

4. While the chicken is baking, prepare the sauce by mixing honey, coconut aminos, and rosemary in a small saucepan over medium-low heat. Bring to a simmer, then reduce the heat to low and simmer for 10 minutes.

5. Divide the mixed greens and chicken among four plates. Drizzle with the honey sauce. Serve hot.

6. Store leftovers in an airtight container in the refrigerator for up to 3 to 4 days.

Per Serving: Calories: 501; Total Fat: 14g; Total Carbs: 34g; Fiber: 3g; Net Carbs: 31g; Protein: 57g

Turkey Cutlets with Cranberry Glaze and Mashed Cauliflower

SERVES 4 / PREP TIME: 5 MINUTES / COOK TIME: 20 MINUTES

This tasty dinner almost feels like a Thanksgiving meal, but without all the time and effort. We love the sweet and savory combination in this recipe. Make a double batch and enjoy it as leftovers throughout the week.

4 (6-ounce) turkey cutlets

1 teaspoon pink Himalayan salt or sea salt

¼ teaspoon garlic powder

1 cup fresh or frozen cranberries

2 tablespoons raw honey

2 tablespoons filtered water

2 tablespoons freshly squeezed orange juice

2 tablespoons red wine vinegar

¼ cup coconut sugar

1 recipe Cauliflower Mash (page 189)

Make It Easier: For a simpler method and less cleanup, use an immersion blender to blend the cranberries while they are right in the pan.

1. Preheat the oven to 400°F. Line a large baking sheet with parchment paper.

2. Season the turkey cutlets on both sides with salt and garlic powder. Place the turkey on the baking sheet and bake for about 20 minutes.

3. While the turkey is baking, prepare the sauce by putting the cranberries, honey, water, orange juice, vinegar, and coconut sugar in a medium saucepan over medium heat. Bring to a boil and boil for about 10 minutes. Transfer to a blender and blend until the sauce is smooth. The liquids will be hot, so place a dish towel over the top of the blender lid before turning it on.

4. Divide the turkey cutlets among four plates and top with sauce. Serve hot alongside the cauliflower mash.

5. Store leftovers in an airtight container in the refrigerator for up to 3 to 4 days.

Per Serving: Calories: 429; Total Fat: 14g; Total Carbs: 33g; Fiber: 4g; Net Carbs: 29g; Protein: 43g

Roasted Duck Breasts with Mashed Sweet Potatoes

SERVES 4 / PREP TIME: 10 MINUTES / COOK TIME: 25 MINUTES

The key to this elegant and anti-inflammatory meal is rendering the duck fat and crisping the skin. Add the rendered duck fat to the mashed sweet potatoes to make them extra smooth and delicious.

2 large sweet potatoes, peeled and chopped into large pieces

4 duck breast fillets

Pink Himalayan salt or sea salt

1 cup seedless red grapes

¼ teaspoon dried thyme or 1 teaspoon chopped fresh thyme

½ cup reserved duck fat

¼ cup pure maple syrup

1. Preheat the oven to 400°F.

2. Place a steamer basket inside a large pot and fill with just enough filtered water to reach the bottom of the basket. Place the sweet potato pieces in the basket and set the heat to high to bring the water to a boil. Reduce the heat, cover, and steam for 15 to 20 minutes, or until tender.

3. While the sweet potatoes are steaming, prepare the duck breasts. With a sharp knife, score the fat of the duck breasts in a crisscross pattern and season the duck with salt.

4. Heat a large cast iron or oven-safe skillet over medium heat. Place the duck fat-side down to render the fat, about 6 minutes. Use a spoon to carefully transfer the duck fat to a small bowl. Set aside.

5. Flip the duck and sear for 1 minute, then add the grapes to the skillet. Turn the breasts to fat-side down again and transfer the skillet to the oven. Roast for 10 minutes, or until the internal temperature reaches 140°F for medium. Rest for 5 minutes before slicing thinly.

6. While the duck is resting, finish the mashed sweet potatoes. In a food processor or blender, or just using a handheld potato masher and a large bowl, combine the steamed sweet potatoes, thyme, reserved duck fat, maple syrup, and salt. Pulse or mash until smooth. Serve hot alongside the sliced duck breast.

7. Store leftovers in an airtight container in the refrigerator for up to 3 to 4 days.

Ingredient Spotlight: Duck fat contains zinc and selenium, which can help boost your immune system. The antioxidants can also help destroy free radicals and remove them from your body.

Per Serving: Calories: 534; Total Fat: 32g; Total Carbs: 33g; Fiber: 2g; Net Carbs: 31g; Protein: 29g

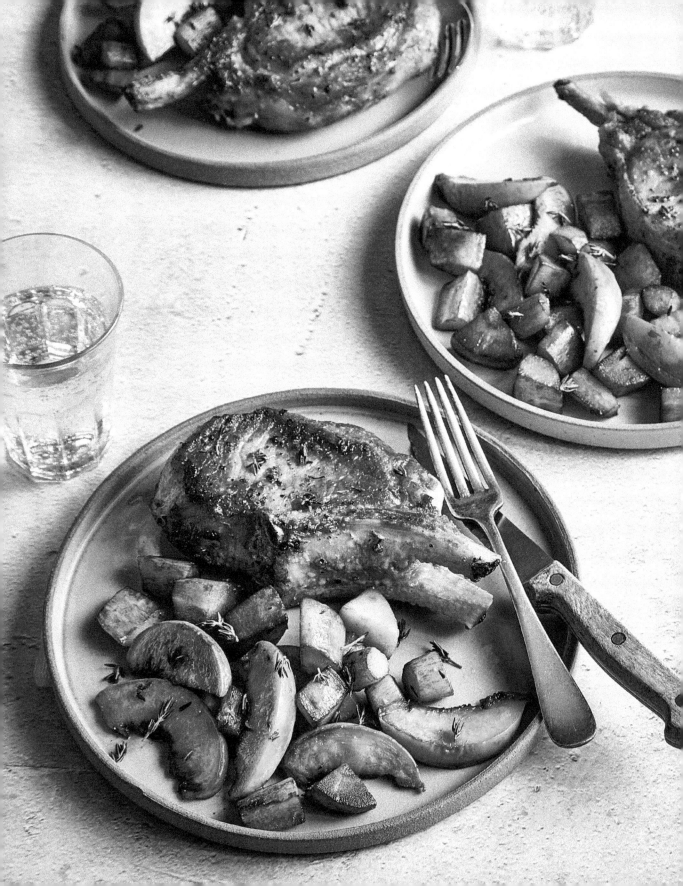

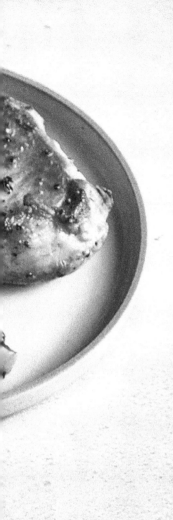

Pork Chops with Peaches and Parsnips *page 146*

Egg Roll in a Bowl

This egg roll in a bowl recipe is one is the easiest dinners in this book. It has all the good things you find inside an egg roll, without the wrapper. Our version has tons of flavor and you can eat it during the AIP-elimination phase. Make a large batch so you can enjoy the leftovers.

2 tablespoons avocado oil

½ cup diced yellow onion

2 garlic cloves, minced

2 teaspoons grated fresh ginger

1½ pounds ground pork

1 teaspoon pink Himalayan salt or sea salt

1 (14-ounce) bag coleslaw mix

3 tablespoons coconut aminos

1 tablespoon white wine vinegar

1. In a large skillet, heat the oil over medium heat. Add the onion, garlic, and ginger, and sauté for 2 to 3 minutes. Add the pork and salt and stir to combine. Cook 6 to 8 minutes, until the pork is cooked through.

2. Stir in the coleslaw mix, coconut aminos, and vinegar.

3. Cook for an additional 3 to 5 minutes, or until the slaw has softened but is still crisp. Serve hot in bowls.

4. Store leftovers in an airtight container in the refrigerator for up to 3 to 4 days.

Swap or Substitute: For a smokier, more savory flavor, replace the avocado oil with an equal amount of sesame oil, if you have reintroduced seeds.

Per Serving: Calories: 312; Total Fat: 14g; Total Carbs: 9g; Fiber: 3g; Net Carbs: 6g; Protein: 39g

Sticky Pork Meatballs with Shirataki Rice

SERVES 4 / PREP TIME: 10 MINUTES / COOK TIME: 20 MINUTES

These meatballs are sweet and sticky and perfect for any night of the week. If you have reintroduced seeds, add a tablespoon of sesame oil to the sauce and garnish with sesame seeds.

2 (7-ounce) packages shirataki rice

1 pound ground pork

1 small onion, grated

1 garlic clove, minced

1 teaspoon grated fresh ginger

1 teaspoon pink Himalayan salt or sea salt

5 tablespoons coconut aminos, divided

2½ tablespoons fish sauce, divided

2 tablespoons raw honey

Make It Easier: To create smooth meatballs, rub your hands with olive oil before rolling them into balls.

1. Prepare the shirataki rice according to package instructions. Set aside.

2. Preheat the oven to 400°F. Line a large baking sheet with parchment paper.

3. In a large bowl, combine the pork, onion, garlic, ginger, 1 tablespoon of coconut aminos, ½ tablespoon of fish sauce, and salt. Roll into 1½-inch meatballs and place on the baking sheet. Bake for 15 to 20 minutes, or until cooked through.

4. While the meatballs are cooking, prepare the sauce by combining the remaining 4 tablespoons of coconut aminos, remaining 2 tablespoons of fish sauce, and honey in a medium saucepan over medium-low heat. Bring to a simmer, then reduce the heat to low and simmer for 10 minutes.

5. Toss the meatballs in with the sauce and stir until well coated. Divide the shirataki rice among four shallow bowls. Top with the meatballs. Serve hot.

6. Store leftovers in an airtight container in the refrigerator for up to 3 to 4 days.

Per Serving: Calories: 195; Total Fat: 5g; Total Carbs: 12g; Fiber: 1g; Net Carbs: 11g; Protein: 27g

Glazed Pork Tenderloin with Roasted Pineapple

SERVES 4 / PREP TIME: 5 MINUTES
MARINATE TIME: 4 HOURS / COOK TIME: 30 MINUTES

Sweet and savory come together in this quick and easy anti-inflammatory dinner. When you're buying canned pineapple, avoid anything that's canned in heavy syrup, which is basically thick sugar water. Look for organic pineapple canned in nothing but pineapple juice (such as Native Forest brand). Drain off the juice and drink it as you cook—or use it instead of water in the recipe.

¼ cup avocado oil

½ cup coconut aminos

2 garlic cloves, minced

2 teaspoons grated fresh ginger

1 pound boneless pork tenderloin

1 teaspoon pink Himalayan salt or sea salt

¼ cup filtered water

1 (15- to 20-ounce) can pineapple slices packed in 100-percent pineapple juice, drained

1. In a large shallow glass dish, whisk together the avocado oil, coconut aminos, garlic, and ginger. Rub the pork all over with salt, then place it in the marinade and turn to coat it on all sides. Cover with plastic wrap and refrigerate to marinate for at least 4 hours.

2. Preheat the oven to 425°F. Line a baking sheet with aluminum foil.

3. Place the pork on the baking sheet and bake for 25 minutes, until the pork is cooked through but still has a slightly pinkish color, or until the internal temperature reaches 135° to 140°F.

4. While the pork is cooking, pour the remaining marinade plus the water into a small saucepan set over medium heat. Bring the sauce to a boil and cook for 5 minutes, then reduce the heat to low and simmer for 5 minutes, or until thickened.

5. Remove pork from the oven and rest on a cutting board. The temperature should rise to 145°F.

6. Set an oven rack 4 to 5 inches from the heat source and turn on the broiler. Place the pineapple rings on the lined baking sheet you used for the pork, and broil for 3 to 5 minutes, or until brown on top.

7. Cut the pork into slices and pour the sauce over them. Serve alongside the pineapple rings.

8. Store leftovers in an airtight container in the refrigerator for up to 3 to 4 days.

Swap or Substitute: If you want to use a fresh pineapple and make your own rings, cut off the top and bottom with a sharp knife. Use the knife to cut the skin off, making sure to cut off all the spiky "eyes." Lay the pineapple on its side and cut it into ¾-inch rings. Finally, use a 1- to 2-inch round cookie cutter or knife to cut out the center core.

Per Serving: Calories: 332; Total Fat: 18g; Total Carbs: 16g; Fiber: 1g; Net Carbs: 15g; Protein: 28g

Pork Chops with Peaches and Parsnips

SERVES 4 / PREP TIME: 5 MINUTES / COOK TIME: 20 MINUTES

Pork chops are a great option when you want a hearty dinner but want it quickly and with minimal effort. We love how the sweet peaches really complement the pork and how the roasted parsnips complete the whole meal.

1 pound parsnips, peeled and roughly chopped

¼ teaspoon garlic powder

½ teaspoon pink Himalayan salt or sea salt, plus 1 teaspoon

4 bone-in pork chops

½ cup balsamic vinegar

1 tablespoon raw honey

1 teaspoon dried thyme or 1 tablespoon chopped fresh thyme

2 tablespoons extra-virgin olive oil

2 peaches, sliced

Ingredient Spotlight: Peaches contain a good amount of soluble fiber, which becomes food for the beneficial bacteria in your intestines. These bacteria produce short-chain fatty acids, which can reduce inflammation in your gut and ease the symptoms of autoimmune diseases.

1. Bring a large pot of salted filtered water to a boil. Add the parsnips, cover, and cook for 15 minutes. Drain and toss with the garlic powder and ½ teaspoon salt.

2. While the parsnips are cooking, prepare the pork chops. Season them on both sides with 1 teaspoon salt. Preheat the broiler and set a large ovenproof skillet over medium-high heat.

3. In a small bowl, whisk together the vinegar, honey, and thyme. Set aside.

4. Heat the oil in the skillet, then add the pork chops and sear for 3 minutes on each side. Reduce the heat to medium and continue to cook for 5 to 8 minutes, or until almost cooked but still pink inside. Add the parsnips.

5. Pour the sauce over the pork chops and parsnips, and toss to coat. Add the peach slices and put the skillet under the broiler for 4 minutes, until brown and crispy. Serve hot.

6. Store leftovers in an airtight container in the refrigerator for up to 3 to 4 days.

Per Serving: Calories: 445; Total Fat: 14g; Total Carbs: 38g; Fiber: 7g; Net Carbs: 31g; Protein: 41g

Creamy Angel Hair Shirataki Noodles with Italian Meat Sauce

SERVES 4 / PREP TIME: 10 MINUTES / COOK TIME: 25 MINUTES

This anti-inflammatory dinner is our take on classic Italian spaghetti with meat sauce. Easy and filling, you'll love making this delicious dish any night of the week. Make a double batch of the meatballs and sauce and freeze the extras so you have an easy dinner ready to go with minimal effort. You can also serve this over cauliflower rice or steamed cauliflower or broccoli.

3 (7-ounce) packages angel hair shirataki noodles

½ pound ground beef

½ pound ground pork

1½ teaspoons pink Himalayan salt or sea salt, divided

½ teaspoon garlic powder

½ teaspoon dried oregano

1 tablespoon coconut aminos

1½ cups "Nomato" Sauce (page 184)

½ cup full-fat unsweetened coconut milk (store-bought or homemade, page 174)

1. Prepare the shirataki noodles according to the package instruction. Set aside.

2. In a large bowl, mix the beef, pork, 1 teaspoon of salt, garlic powder, oregano, and coconut aminos.

3. Transfer the mixture to a large skillet and cook, breaking it up and stirring often, until browned, 6 to 8 minutes. Reduce the heat to medium low and add the "Nomato" Sauce, coconut milk, and ½ teaspoon of salt.

4. Simmer for 5 minutes, then add the cooked shirataki noodles. Cook for an additional 10 minutes. Serve hot.

5. Store leftovers in an airtight container in the refrigerator for up to 3 to 4 days.

Swap or Substitute: The ground beef and ground pork can be replaced with 1 pound of ground chicken or turkey. Or mix several types of ground meat, so you end up with 1 pound of ground meat.

Per Serving: Calories: 256; Total Fat: 14g; Total Carbs: 9g; Fiber: 2g; Net Carbs: 7g; Protein: 26g

Bacon-Wrapped Meatloaf with Roasted Brussels Sprouts

SERVES 4 / PREP TIME: 5 MINUTES / COOK TIME: 55 MINUTES

This American classic has all the flavors that you know and love but with all anti-inflammatory ingredients. It cooks for a while, but there is very little prep time, so you basically just pop it in the oven. Serve it with our "Nomato" Sauce (page 184) or our Classic Ranch Dressing (page 178) to make it even tastier.

½ pound ground beef

½ pound ground pork

1 small onion, finely diced

2 garlic cloves, minced

¼ teaspoon dried thyme or 1 teaspoon chopped fresh thyme

1½ teaspoon pink Himalayan salt or sea salt, divided

1 tablespoon coconut aminos

8 slices uncooked bacon

1 pound Brussels sprouts, cut in half or quartered

1 tablespoon avocado oil

Swap or Substitute:
Add ¼ teaspoon of freshly ground black pepper to the meatloaf, if you have successfully reintroduced it.

1. Preheat the oven to 400°F. Line a large baking sheet with parchment paper.

2. In a large bowl, use your hands to mix together the beef, pork, onion, garlic, thyme, 1 teaspoon of salt, and coconut aminos. Transfer the mixture to a medium loaf pan and press it evenly into the pan. Arrange the bacon on top.

3. Bake for about 30 minutes on the center rack of the oven.

4. While the meatloaf is baking, prepare the Brussels sprouts by tossing them with the oil and remaining ½ teaspoon of salt on the baking sheet. After the meatloaf has baked for 30 minutes, put the Brussels sprouts in the oven on the top rack and cook for another for 20 to 25 minutes, until they're starting to brown and crisp and the internal temperature on the meat-loaf reaches 165°F.

5. Slice the meatloaf and serve alongside the Brussels sprouts.

6. Store leftovers in an airtight container in the refrigerator for up to 3 to 4 days.

Per Serving: Calories: 446; Total Fat: 29g; Total Carbs: 13g; Fiber: 5g; Net Carbs: 8g; Protein: 35g

Shepherd's Pie

Shepherd's pie is comfort food at its best! Our version features a hearty beef-and-vegetable layer topped with creamy cauliflower mash. This dish is a perfect reason to make a big batch of cauliflower mash on the weekend, and then use it in dishes all week. If you don't have any, just toss ½ pound of cauliflower florets with a little avocado oil and salt and roast it in a parchment paper–lined baking pan while you bake the topless pie. Serve the roasted cauliflower on top of or next to the meat.

2 tablespoons avocado oil

1 yellow onion, diced

6 garlic cloves, minced

1 pound ground lamb

1 pound ground beef

1 cup chopped frozen carrots

¼ cup coconut aminos

¼ cup balsamic vinegar

1 tablespoon dried oregano

Pinch pink Himalayan salt or sea salt

1 recipe Cauliflower Mash (page 189)

Swap or Substitute: Use 2 pounds of ground beef in the recipe if you don't like lamb. Or use a mixture of ground beef, turkey, pork, and/or chicken.

1. Preheat the oven to 425°F.

2. Heat the avocado oil in a large skillet over medium-high heat. Add the onion and garlic and sauté, stirring constantly, until softened, about 5 minutes. Add the lamb and beef and cook for an additional 5 to 7 minutes.

3. When the meat is almost done cooking, add the carrots, coconut aminos, vinegar, oregano, and salt. Stir to combine and cook for another 3 to 5 minutes.

4. Transfer the meat mixture to a 9-inch pie plate and spread in an even layer. Top with the cauliflower mash. Use a spatula to spread out the mashed cauliflower evenly in one layer.

5. Bake on the top rack of the oven for 10 to 15 minutes, until heated through and the top starts to brown.

6. Store any leftovers in an airtight container in the refrigerator for up to 3 to 4 days.

Per Serving: Calories: 453; Total Fat: 29g; Total Carbs: 15g; Fiber: 4g; Net Carbs: 11g; Protein: 36g

Greek Meatball and Zucchini Noodle Bowls

SERVES 4 / PREP TIME: 10 MINUTES / COOK TIME: 15 MINUTES

This dish is so easy because the meatballs and zucchini noodles cook in the oven at the same temperature. Use packaged zucchini noodles to speed up the prep time. To make smooth meatballs, rub your hands with oil before rolling the meat mixture. This will keep the meat from sticking to your hands.

½ pound ground beef

½ pound ground lamb

½ medium red onion, grated

2 tablespoons finely chopped fresh mint

1 garlic clove, minced

1 tablespoon coconut aminos

1 teaspoon pink Himalayan salt or sea salt

1 teaspoon dried oregano or 1 tablespoon finely chopped fresh oregano

2 zucchini, spiralized or cut into noodles

¼ cup Classic Ranch Dressing (page 178)

Ingredient Spotlight: Zucchini noodles tend to produce liquid when heated. If that matters to you, dry them by letting them sit between two layers of paper towels for 15 minutes. or let them air-dry for 30 minutes.

1. Preheat the oven to 400°F. Line two baking sheets with parchment paper.

2. In a large bowl, use your hands to mix together the beef, lamb, onion, mint, garlic, coconut aminos, salt, and oregano. Be careful not to overmix. Form the mixture into 1½-inch balls and place on one of the baking sheets. Bake for about 15 minutes, or until the internal temperature reaches 160°F.

3. Place the zucchini noodles on the other baking sheet. Put them in the oven during the last 5 minutes of cooking the meatballs, just to heat through.

4. Divide the zucchini noodles among 4 plates, drizzle with ranch dressing, and top with the meatballs. Serve hot.

5. Store leftovers in an airtight container in the refrigerator for up to 3 to 4 days.

Per Serving: Calories: 241; Total Fat: 12g; Total Carbs: 5g; Fiber: 1g; Net Carbs: 4g; Protein: 26g

Sloppy Joe Casserole

SERVES 4 / PREP TIME: 5 MINUTES / COOK TIME: 40 MINUTES

This meaty and hearty dinner is sure to be a crowd pleaser with kids and adults alike. To make this delicious meal even easier, make a double batch of our "Nomato" Sauce (page 184) ahead of time so that it is ready to use in a variety of recipes.

1 pound ground beef

1 onion, diced

½ teaspoon garlic powder

1½ teaspoons pink Himalayan salt or sea salt, divided

1½ cups "Nomato" Sauce (page 184)

1 (1-pound) bag cauliflower rice

1 garlic clove, minced

3 tablespoons lard

2 teaspoons fish sauce

2 teaspoons apple cider vinegar

1. Preheat the oven to 350°F.

2. In a large skillet over medium heat, combine the beef, onion, garlic powder, and 1 teaspoon of salt. Cook about 5 minutes, until the beef is almost cooked through, then add the sauce. Reduce the heat to low and simmer for 10 minutes while you prepare the cauliflower mixture.

3. In a 9-by-11-inch casserole dish, mix the cauliflower rice with the garlic, lard, fish sauce, apple cider vinegar, and remaining ½ teaspoon salt. Smooth it over the bottom of the dish. Smooth the meat sauce over the cauliflower layer.

4. Bake for about 20 minutes, or until the casserole is heated through. Serve hot.

5. Store leftovers in an airtight container in the refrigerator for up to 3 to 4 days.

Swap or Substitute: Replace the lard with butter if you have successfully reintroduced it.

Per Serving: Calories: 332; Total Fat: 19g; Total Carbs: 16g; Fiber: 5g; Net Carbs: 11g; Protein: 28g

Pan-Seared Filet Mignon with Arugula Salad

SERVES 4 / PREP TIME: 5 MINUTES
COOK TIME: 9 MINUTES / REST TIME: 10 MINUTES

Re-create a steakhouse experience with this delicious and simple recipe. Serve it with our AIP Garlic Herb Flatbread (page 62) for an even more filling meal.

4 (10-ounce) filet mignon steaks, about 2 inches thick, at room temperature

2 teaspoons pink Himalayan salt or sea salt

¼ teaspoon garlic powder

2 tablespoons lard

½ teaspoon dried thyme or 1½ teaspoons chopped fresh thyme

4 cups arugula

3 tablespoons Balsamic Vinaigrette (page 176)

Swap or Substitute:
Replace the lard with butter, if you have successfully reintroduced it. The thyme can be replaced with equal amounts of rosemary.

1. Preheat the oven to 400°F.

2. Season the steaks with salt and garlic powder. Set a large ovenproof skillet over high heat and melt the lard. Sprinkle the thyme into the melted lard. Place the steaks in the hot skillet and sear for 2 minutes on each side.

3. Transfer the skillet to the oven to bake for 5 minutes for medium rare, or until the internal temperature reaches 120°F. Or cook them longer, depending on how you like your steak, using a meat thermometer to determine doneness.

4. Remove the skillet from the oven and rest the steaks for 10 minutes. They will continue to cook and reach 130°F.

5. While the steaks are resting, toss the arugula and dressing together in a large bowl.

6. Serve warm with salad on the side. This is best eaten right away.

Per Serving: Calories: 944; Total Fat: 75g; Total Carbs: 3g; Fiber: 0g; Net Carbs: 3g; Protein: 52g

Chimichurri Skirt Steak with Avocado Salad

SERVES 4 / PREP TIME: 10 MINUTES / MARINATE TIME: 4 TO 8 HOURS
COOK TIME: 10 MINUTES / REST TIME: 10 MINUTES

The marinating time might seem intimidating, but throwing together the marinade and popping the steak in the refrigerator only takes 5 minutes. Chimichurri keeps in the refrigerator, so just pull out the jar you made over the weekend to finish the dish. And always remember to cut skirt steaks against the grain.

2 tablespoons avocado oil

Juice of ½ lemon

2 garlic cloves, minced

½ teaspoon dried oregano

½ teaspoon pink Himalayan salt or sea salt

1¼ pounds skirt steak

½ cup Chimichurri (page 182)

2 avocados, pitted, peeled, and chopped

3 tablespoons Chimichurri (page 182)

Ingredient Spotlight: Skirt steaks are one of our favorite cuts of beef because their rich flavor can stand up to a sauce. But they can be a little tough, which is why marinating the steak for at least 4 hours is crucial to allow the acid in the marinade to break down the proteins in the meat and tenderize it.

1. Combine the avocado oil, lemon juice, garlic, oregano, and salt in a shallow dish. Pat the steak dry with a paper towel and place it in the marinade. Flip to coat both sides. Cover and marinate in the refrigerator for 4 to 8 hours.

2. Heat the grill or a stovetop grill pan to high.

3. Cook the steak for 3 to 6 minutes on each side, or until the internal temperature reaches 120°F for medium rare. Or cook them longer, depending on how you like your steak, using a meat thermometer to determine doneness. Remove the steak from the heat and rest for about 10 minutes. It will continue to cook and reach 130°F.

4. While the steak rests, gently toss the avocado and chimichurri together in a medium bowl until combined.

5. Cut the steak against the grain. Drizzle with the chimichurri and serve immediately alongside the avocado salad.

Per Serving: Calories: 567; Total Fat: 43g; Total Carbs: 14g; Fiber: 9g; Net Carbs: 5g; Protein: 34g

Reverse-Seared Rib Eyes with Spinach Salad

SERVES 4 / PREP TIME: 5 MINUTES
COOK TIME: 20 MINUTES / REST TIME: 10 MINUTES

A reverse sear means cooking the steaks in the oven at a relatively low temperature, then searing the outside in a very hot skillet. This gives the steaks a beautiful crust and keeps the inside evenly cooked.

FOR THE STEAKS

4 (6-ounce) rib eye steaks, room temperature

2 teaspoons pink Himalayan salt or sea salt

½ teaspoon garlic powder

2 tablespoons avocado oil

1 teaspoon dried rosemary or 2 sprigs fresh rosemary

FOR THE SPINACH SALAD

6 cups baby spinach

2 red radishes, thinly sliced

1 carrot, grated

2 tablespoons salad dressing of your choice (see chapter 10)

Swap or Substitute: You can replace the rosemary with an equal amount of thyme.

1. Preheat the oven to 275°F. Place a large oven-proof skillet in the oven. Set a wire cooking rack on top of a large baking sheet.

2. Season the steaks with salt and garlic powder on both sides. Place them on the rack and bake for 15 minutes, or until the internal temperature reaches 90°F. Carefully remove the steaks and the skillet.

3. Place the skillet on the stovetop over high heat. Pour the avocado oil in the skillet, then add the rosemary. Sear the steaks for 1 to 2 minutes on each side, or until the internal temperature reaches 120°F for medium rare. Or cook them longer, depending on how you like your steak, using a meat thermometer to determine doneness.

4. Rest the steaks for 10 minutes. They will continue to cook and reach 130°F.

5. TO MAKE THE SPINACH SALAD: Divide the spinach, radish, and carrot across four plates, and drizzle dressing over each. Plate the rib eyes alongside the salads. These steaks are best eaten right away.

Per Serving: Calories: 446; Total Fat: 28g; Total Carbs: 14g; Fiber: 4g; Net Carbs: 10g; Protein: 36g

Beef Tenderloin with Garlic Mushrooms

SERVES 4 / PREP TIME: 5 MINUTES
COOK TIME: 30 MINUTES / REST TIME: 15 MINUTES

This elegant dish is perfect for dinner parties or fancy nights in—but it also makes a comforting meal when you're craving a hearty, filling dish. Let the oven do the majority of the work in this recipe, which can easily be doubled.

FOR THE BEEF TENDERLOIN

1¼ pounds boneless beef tenderloin, at room temperature

1 tablespoon avocado oil

2 teaspoons pink Himalayan salt or sea salt

½ teaspoon dried thyme, or 2 teaspoons chopped fresh thyme

½ teaspoon garlic powder

FOR THE GARLIC MUSHROOMS

1 pound cremini mushrooms

1 teaspoon dried thyme, or 1 tablespoon chopped fresh thyme

2 garlic cloves, minced

2 tablespoons avocado oil

¾ teaspoon pink Himalayan salt or sea salt

1. Preheat the oven to 425°F. Line a large baking sheet with parchment paper.

2. Heat a large ovenproof skillet over high heat. Rub the beef on both sides with avocado oil and sprinkle with salt, thyme, and garlic powder. Sear about 2 minutes on each side.

3. Transfer the skillet to the middle rack of the oven. Cook for about 25 minutes, or until the internal temperature reaches 120°F for medium rare. Remove from the oven and rest for 15 minutes. It will continue to cook and reach 130°F.

4. TO MAKE THE GARLIC MUSHROOMS: Toss the mushrooms, thyme, garlic, oil, and salt together on the baking sheet. Bake in the oven along with the beef for 15 minutes.

5. Slice the beef and serve immediately alongside the mushrooms.

Ingredient Spotlight: Mushrooms contain selenium and are one of the few foods that contain vitamin D.

Per Serving: Calories: 507; Total Fat: 41g; Total Carbs: 5g; Fiber: 2g; Net Carbs: 3g; Protein: 28g

Slow Cooker Short Ribs with Cauliflower Rice

SERVES 4 / PREP TIME: 10 MINUTES / COOK TIME: 6 TO 8 HOURS

Slow cooker meals are perfect for days when you want to come home to a dinner that's already cooked and waiting for you. Chop and prep everything the night before, then just sear the ribs in the morning (4 minutes!) and throw everything else in the slow cooker. Freeze the extra short ribs and enjoy them whenever you need a quick meal with minimal effort.

3 pounds bone-in short ribs

1 teaspoon pink Himalayan salt or sea salt

1 tablespoon avocado oil

4 medium carrots, cut into 1½-inch pieces

3 cups beef broth or beef bone broth (store-bought or homemade, page 191)

2 tablespoons apple cider vinegar

1 tablespoon dried thyme or 6 sprigs fresh thyme

2 onions, roughly chopped

6 garlic cloves, minced

1 (1-pound) bag cauliflower rice

1. Season the short ribs all over with salt.

2. Heat the avocado oil in a large skillet over medium heat. Cook the short ribs for 1 to 2 minutes on each side. Transfer to a 4- or 5-quart slow cooker. Add the carrots, broth, vinegar, thyme, onions, and garlic.

3. Cook, covered, on low for 6 to 8 hours or until the meat is tender.

4. Add the cauliflower rice during the last hour of cooking and stir to combine. Serve warm.

5. Store leftovers in an airtight container in the refrigerator for up to 4 days.

Ingredient Spotlight: Do not skip searing the short ribs. This step is crucial for the ribs to develop their flavors and helps break down the proteins, resulting in more tender meat.

Per Serving: Calories: 976; Total Fat: 65g; Total Carbs: 26g; Fiber: 6g; Net Carbs: 20g; Protein: 76g

Rosemary Lamb Chops with Honey-Roasted Carrots

SERVES 4 / PREP TIME: 5 MINUTES / COOK TIME: 45 MINUTES

If you are getting bored of chicken and beef, switch it up and make these delicious and noninflammatory lamb chops. Make the carrots in the oven first, then turn on the broiler to cook the lamb chops.

FOR THE CARROTS

1 (1-pound) bag baby carrots

1 tablespoon avocado oil

1 tablespoon raw honey

½ teaspoon dried rosemary, or 2 teaspoons chopped fresh rosemary

½ teaspoon pink Himalayan salt or sea salt

FOR THE LAMB CHOPS

12 lamb rib chops

1 tablespoon avocado oil

1 teaspoon pink Himalayan salt or sea salt

1 teaspoon dried rosemary, or 1 tablespoon chopped fresh rosemary

¼ teaspoon garlic powder

1. Preheat the oven to 400°F. Line a baking sheet with parchment paper. Move an oven rack to 4 to 5 inches below the heat source for the broiler.

2. Place the carrots on the baking sheet and toss with avocado oil, honey, vinegar, rosemary, and salt. Bake for 35 to 40 minutes, or until the carrots are easily pierced with a fork.

3. TO MAKE THE LAMB CHOPS: Rub them with avocado oil on both sides, then sprinkle with salt, rosemary, and garlic powder. Place in a broiler pan.

4. When the carrots are done, take them out of the oven and turn on the broiler. Broil the lamb chops for about 2½ minutes on each side. The internal temperature should reach 145°F for medium rare.

5. Serve immediately alongside the carrots.

Ingredient Spotlight: Rosemary extract has been shown to fight irritable bowel syndrome and rosemary oil can prevent hair loss, both of which are common complaints among those suffering from autoimmune disease.

Per Serving: Calories: 302; Total Fat: 16g; Total Carbs: 15g; Fiber: 3g; Net Carbs: 12g; Protein: 26g

Bison Burgers with Roasted Zucchini

SERVES 4 / PREP TIME: 10 MINUTES / COOK TIME: 30 MINUTES

Whether you are grilling outdoors or cooking inside, this burger is an interesting alternative to a typical beef burger. The burgers cook super fast; it's the zucchini that needs some time (but the prep for them is 5 minutes or less). You can cook these burgers outside on the grill if you want, 3 to 4 minutes on each side. For a classic summer barbecue presentation, put some arugula on each plate, place a burger on top, and drizzle with Classic Ranch Dressing (page 178).

FOR THE ZUCCHINI

3 medium zucchini, cut into strips

2 tablespoons avocado oil

½ teaspoon garlic powder

½ teaspoon pink Himalayan salt or sea salt

FOR THE BURGERS

1¼ pounds ground bison

2 tablespoons coconut aminos

1 teaspoon pink Himalayan salt or sea salt

¼ teaspoon garlic powder

1 tablespoon avocado oil

TO MAKE THE ZUCCHINI

1. Preheat the oven to 400°F. Line a large baking sheet with parchment paper.

2. Place the zucchini in a large bowl and toss gently with the avocado oil, salt, and garlic powder.

3. Spread out the zucchini on the baking sheet. Bake for 30 minutes, flipping halfway through.

TO MAKE THE BURGERS

4. When zucchini is almost done, prepare the burgers. In a large bowl, combine the bison, coconut aminos, salt, and garlic powder and gently mix well. Form into 4 patties. Rub the avocado oil on the patties to prevent them from sticking.

5. Place a cooking rack over a broiler pan and put the burgers on the rack.

6. Remove the zucchini from the oven, and turn on the broiler. Broil the burgers for 3 to 4 minutes, flip, and broil on the other side for 3 to 4 minutes, or until the internal temperature reaches 160°F.

7. Serve hot along with the zucchini. These are best eaten right away.

Ingredient Spotlight: What we sometimes call buffalo are actually bison—a relative of the ox and cow that's native to North America and Europe. Bison are raised commercially for their meat. Bison meat is more likely to be grass-fed, making it perfect for those following an anti-inflammatory diet.

Per Serving: Calories: 331; Total Fat: 21g; Total Carbs: 5g; Fiber: 2g; Net Carbs: 3g; Protein: 31g

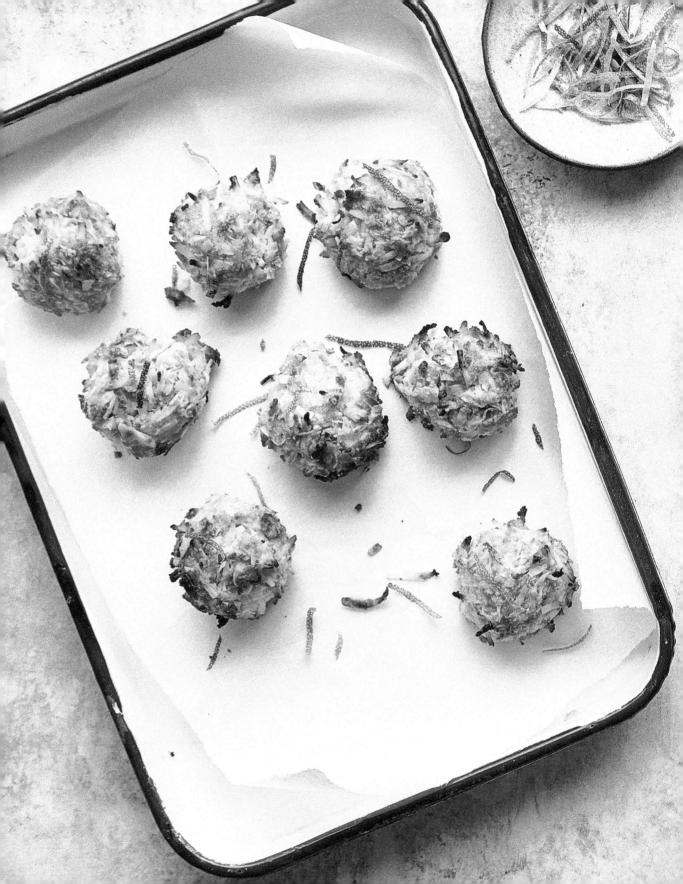

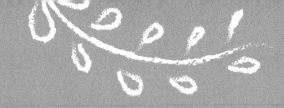

CHAPTER 9

DESSERTS

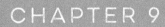

Coconut Lime Macaroons *page 167*

Banana Soft Serve

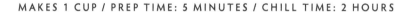

MAKES 1 CUP / PREP TIME: 5 MINUTES / CHILL TIME: 2 HOURS

Whip up this luscious soft-serve treat whenever you want something cold and sweet. It comes together quickly, with only two ingredients, and is a great way to use up bananas before they go bad. Feel free to experiment with optional add-ins, such as cinnamon, carob powder, or ginger.

1 ripe banana, peeled and sliced into circles

1 teaspoon raw honey

1. Arrange the banana slices in a single layer on a baking sheet in a single layer and transfer to the freezer for at least 2 hours.

2. Put the frozen banana slices and honey in a blender or food processor. Process until smooth. Serve cold.

Make It Easier: If you aren't planning to use the frozen banana slices immediately, transfer them to an airtight container in the freezer so that they don't get freezer burn. They will keep for about 1 month.

Per Serving: Calories: 127; Total Fat: 0g; Total Carbs: 33g; Fiber: 3g; Net Carbs: 30g; Protein: 1g

Grilled Pineapple

SERVES 6 TO 8 / PREP TIME: 5 MINUTES / COOK TIME: 10 MINUTES

Grilling a pineapple brings out its natural juices and intensifies its sweetness. This easy dessert is one of our very favorites. One bite of this grilled pineapple will immediately transport you to a tropical island. For a guide to cutting a fresh pineapple, see our recipe for Glazed Pork Tenderloin with Roasted Pineapple (page 144). Or you can use 1 (15- to 20-ounce) can of pineapple slices, packed in 100-percent pineapple juice and drained.

2 tablespoons coconut oil

2 teaspoons coconut sugar

½ teaspoon ground cinnamon

1 fresh pineapple, cored and cut into 6 to 8 slices

1. Combine the coconut oil, coconut sugar, and cinnamon in a small bowl.

2. Heat a grill or grill pan to medium-high heat. Grill the pineapple rings for 3 to 5 minutes on each side.

3. Top each grilled pineapple slice with the coconut mixture and enjoy.

4. Store leftovers in an airtight container in the refrigerator for up to 5 days.

Swap or Substitute: If peaches are in season, feel free to use them instead. Just cut three peaches in half and remove the pits. Grill for 7 to 8 minutes on each side.

Per Serving: Calories: 163; Total Fat: 5g; Total Carbs: 32g; Fiber: 3g; Net Carbs: 29g; Protein: 1g

"Chocolate" Pudding

SERVES 4 / PREP TIME: 15 MINUTES

Super creamy and delicious, this is the perfect dessert for when you are craving something chocolaty. Carob makes a great stand-in for chocolate in this no-cook pudding. Make a double batch and refrigerate the extra so you can enjoy it during the week. Use it as a dip for fresh strawberries to make this treat even more special.

⅓ cup coconut sugar

3⅓ cups coconut cream, chilled

⅓ cup carob powder

1 teaspoon vanilla powder

1. Put the coconut sugar in a blender and pulse for 5 to 10 minutes, or until the sugar becomes powdery.

2. Add the coconut cream, carob powder, and vanilla and blend until everything is smooth and fluffy, about 5 minutes.

3. Serve immediately.

4. Store in an airtight container in the refrigerator for up to 7 days.

Swap or Substitute: If you have successfully reintroduced cocoa, substitute ⅓ cup cocoa powder for the carob powder and increase the coconut sugar to ½ cup.

Per Serving: Calories: 745; Total Fat: 70g; Total Carbs: 34g; Fiber: 7g; Net Carbs: 27g; Protein: 9g

Pumpkin Custard

SERVES 4 TO 6 / PREP TIME: 5 MINUTES
COOK TIME: 5 MINUTES / CHILL TIME: 1 TO 2 HOURS

This creamy pumpkin custard is perfect for fall, but also any time of the year when you are craving a cool and delicious treat. Serve with our Coconut Whipped Cream (page 175) and sprinkle with extra cinnamon to make a gorgeous presentation.

1 tablespoon beef gelatin powder

¼ cup warm filtered water

1 cup pumpkin puree

1 cup full-fat unsweetened coconut milk (store-bought or homemade, page 174)

2 teaspoons cinnamon

¼ teaspoon pink Himalayan salt or sea salt

¼ cup coconut sugar

2 teaspoons gluten-free vanilla extract

1. In a small bowl, mix together the gelatin and warm water and let sit, until it forms a gel, about 3 minutes.

2. In a medium saucepan over medium heat, stir together the pumpkin puree, coconut milk, cinnamon, salt, coconut sugar, and vanilla until very hot but not boiling, about 5 minutes. Remove from the heat and slowly stir in the gelatin mixture, whisking until it is dissolved and combined with the pumpkin mixture.

3. Pour the custard into ramekins, small bowls, or glass jars. Refrigerate for 1 to 2 hours, or until firm. Serve cold.

4. Store leftovers in an airtight container in the refrigerator for up to 7 days.

Ingredient Spotlight: To keep a skin from forming on the custard, directly cover the surface with plastic wrap. Be sure there are no air pockets between the custard and the plastic wrap.

Per Serving: Calories: 198; Total Fat: 12g; Total Carbs: 21g; Fiber: 3g; Net Carbs: 18g; Protein: 3g

Coconut Panna Cotta

SERVES 4 / PREP TIME: 5 MINUTES
COOK TIME: 10 MINUTES / CHILL TIME: 4 HOURS

This crave-worthy dessert is a delicious way to sneak beef gelatin into your diet. Gelatin can help ease joint pain, aid in digestive function, and improve skin health. This dessert can be made ahead of time, covered with plastic wrap, and refrigerated for up to 3 to 4 days.

1⅔ cups full-fat unsweetened coconut milk (store-bought or homemade, page 174)

Pinch pink Himalayan salt or sea salt

3 tablespoons raw honey, divided

½ teaspoon gluten-free vanilla extract

1 tablespoon beef gelatin powder

Coconut oil

1. In a medium saucepan, heat the coconut milk, salt, and 2 tablespoons of honey over medium heat for 5 minutes, or until the honey is dissolved. Stir in the vanilla and then turn off the heat. Slowly whisk in the gelatin powder, making sure to break apart any clumps.

2. Grease four ramekins with coconut oil and pour the mixture evenly into the ramekins. Refrigerate for 4 hours, or until set.

3. Dip the ramekins in warm water for 10 seconds to loosen the panna cotta. Place a plate upside down on top of each ramekin, then flip it over. The panna cotta will slide out onto the plate.

4. Drizzle the remaining 1 tablespoon of honey over the four panna cottas before serving.

Ingredient Spotlight: To add extra flavor to this dessert, make a quick warm berry compote by mixing 1 cup of berries and 1 tablespoon of honey in a small saucepan over medium-low heat. Stir constantly for 3 to 5 minutes, or until the berries start to break down, then remove from the heat and pour over top of the panna cottas before serving.

Per Serving: Calories: 240; Total Fat: 20g; Total Carbs: 16g; Fiber: 0g; Net Carbs: 16g; Protein: 3g

Coconut Lime Macaroons

MAKES 10 MACAROONS / PREP TIME: 5 MINUTES / COOK TIME: 10 MINUTES

We love how the coconut and lime combine in these delicious cookies to give a lovely tropical flavor. These cookies are so easy and perfect when you want to whip up a dessert with little effort. For a different twist, replace the lime zest and juice with equal amounts of lemon or orange zest and juice.

1½ cups unsweetened shredded coconut

½ cup coconut butter

2 tablespoons collagen peptides powder

2 tablespoons coconut flour

3 tablespoons raw honey

1½ teaspoons lime zest, plus more for garnish

1 tablespoon lime juice

1. Preheat the oven to 350°F. Line a large baking sheet with parchment paper.

2. In a medium bowl, mix together the shredded coconut, coconut butter, collagen powder, coconut flour, honey, lime zest, and lime juice, using your hands to break apart any clumps. Roll the mixture into 1½-inch balls and place them on the baking sheet.

3. Bake for 10 to 12 minutes, or until the outsides start to brown.

4. Remove from the oven and garnish each cookie with a little extra lime zest. Allow to cool completely before serving.

5. Store leftovers in an airtight container in the refrigerator for up to 7 days.

Ingredient Spotlight: Coconut butter, also known as coconut manna, is the ground-up meat of the coconut. Studies show that the lauric acid found in coconut butter is one of the best ways to strengthen the immune system—second only to a mother's milk.

Per Serving: Calories: 88; Total Fat: 6g; Total Carbs: 8g; Fiber: 1g; Net Carbs: 7g; Protein: 2g

Strawberry Pound Cake

SERVES 12 / PREP TIME: 10 MINUTES / COOK TIME: 30 MINUTES

This is one of our favorite desserts to make for a spring or summer get-together. The pound cake looks so pretty topped with beautiful bright red strawberries fresh from the farmers' market. And for something extra special, top it all with some Coconut Whipped Cream (page 175).

6 tablespoons plus
1 teaspoon coconut oil,
melted and cooled

1 cup tigernut flour

¼ cup cassava flour

2 tablespoons
coconut flour

½ teaspoon baking soda

¼ teaspoon pink
Himalayan salt or sea salt

¼ cup raw honey

2 tablespoons
coconut sugar

1 teaspoon gluten-free
vanilla extract

2 Gelatin Eggs (page 187)

1½ cups roughly
chopped strawberries

1. Preheat the oven to 350°F. Grease a 4-by-8-inch loaf pan with 1 teaspoon of coconut oil and set aside.

2. In a large bowl, mix together the tigernut flour, cassava flour, coconut flour, baking soda, and salt. Add the honey, coconut sugar, remaining 6 table-spoons of coconut oil, and vanilla extract and beat with a handheld electric mixer or a whisk until combined. Add the gelatin eggs to the mixture and beat to combine.

3. Transfer the mixture to the loaf pan. Bake for 25 to 30 minutes, or until the cake is cooked through the center and starting to turn golden brown.

4. Cool on a rack before removing from the loaf pan. Slice the cake and top with strawberries.

5. Store leftover cake and strawberries in separate airtight containers in the refrigerator for up to 7 days. The cake itself will keep in the freezer for up to 3 months.

Swap or Substitute: To switch things up, replace the strawberries with equal amounts of blueberries or raspberries.

Per Serving: Calories: 166; Total Fat: 9g; Total Carbs: 19g; Fiber: 5g; Net Carbs: 14g; Protein: 3g

Snickerdoodle Cookies

MAKES 12 COOKIES / PREP TIME: 15 MINUTES / COOK TIME: 10 MINUTES

We put an anti-inflammatory spin on these classic cinnamon cookies. We love these AIP treats for their delicious flavor and because they are so simple to make. You can always replace the pure maple syrup with equal amounts of raw honey. Make a double batch and freeze half the unbaked dough so that you can make fresh, hot cookies any time.

1 cup tigernut flour

⅔ cup arrowroot starch

¼ cup collagen peptides powder

½ teaspoon baking soda

4 teaspoons cinnamon, divided

¼ teaspoon pink Himalayan salt or sea salt

½ cup coconut oil, melted and cooled

¼ cup pure maple syrup

1 teaspoon apple cider vinegar

1 teaspoon gluten-free vanilla extract

2 tablespoons coconut sugar

Ingredient Spotlight: Using collagen in baking is a great way to get the cookies to hold together and makes a great replacement for eggs.

1. Preheat the oven to 350°F. Line a large baking sheet with parchment paper.

2. In a large bowl, combine the tigernut flour, arrowroot starch, collagen powder, baking soda, 2 teaspoons of cinnamon, and salt. Mix until well combined. Add the coconut oil, maple syrup, vinegar, and vanilla extract and beat until combined.

3. In a small bowl, mix together the coconut sugar and the remaining 2 teaspoons of cinnamon.

4. Use a spoon to scoop out about 1½ tablespoons of dough, then roll into a ball and place on the baking sheet. Lightly press down so it flattens into a thin disk. You should have 12 cookies.

5. Bake for 8 to 10 minutes, or until the edges begin to turn golden brown. Cool on the baking sheet before serving.

6. Store baked cookies in an airtight container at room temperature for up 7 days. Store raw dough in an airtight container in the freezer for up to 3 months.

Per Serving: Calories: 191; Total Fat: 11g; Total Carbs: 20g; Fiber: 4g; Net Carbs: 16g; Protein: 2g

"Noatmeal" Cookies

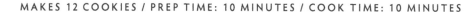

MAKES 12 COOKIES / PREP TIME: 10 MINUTES / COOK TIME: 10 MINUTES

Nothing beats a fresh batch of cookies baking in the oven and the sweet scent of cinnamon throughout your home. These smell and taste of these delicious treats will immediately bring back memories of this childhood classic cookie.

½ cup shredded coconut

½ cup tigernut flour

2 tablespoons cassava flour

1 tablespoon coconut flour

¼ teaspoon baking powder

1 teaspoon cinnamon

2 tablespoons pure maple syrup

1 tablespoon coconut sugar

3 tablespoons coconut oil, melted

1 Gelatin Egg (page 187)

1. Preheat the oven to 375°F. Line a large baking sheet with parchment paper.

2. In a large bowl, combine the shredded coconut, tigernut flour, cassava flour, coconut flour, baking soda, cinnamon, maple syrup, coconut sugar, and coconut oil. Stir until combined. Add the gelatin egg and immediately combine into the mixture.

3. Use a soup spoon to scoop out 1½ tablespoons of dough, then roll into a ball and place on the baking sheet. Lightly press down with your hand so it flattens into a disk. You should have 12 cookies.

4. Bake for 8 to 10 minutes, or until the tops start to turn golden brown. Cool on the baking sheet for at least 10 minutes before serving.

5. Store leftover cookies in an airtight container in the refrigerator for up to 1 week.

Make It Easier: You can store extra baked cookies in an airtight container in the freezer for up to 3 months. To defrost, simply let the cookies sit at room temperature for 30 minutes.

Per Serving: Calories: 96; Total Fat: 5g; Total Carbs: 9g; Fiber: 3g; Net Carbs: 2g; Protein: 1g

Soft Carrot Cake Cookies

Ultra-soft and bursting with the warming flavors of cinnamon and maple syrup, these cookies are super easy and delicious. The carrots keep them extra moist and add a few more nutrients than your typical cookie. This is our favorite cookie to make when we are low on energy but still in the mood for a treat.

½ cup grated carrot

½ cup tigernut flour

2 tablespoons cassava flour

1 tablespoon coconut flour

¼ teaspoon baking powder

1 teaspoon cinnamon

2 tablespoons pure maple syrup

1 tablespoon coconut sugar

3 tablespoons coconut oil, melted

1 Gelatin Egg (page 187)

1. Preheat the oven to 375°F. Line a large baking sheet with parchment paper.

2. In a large bowl, combine the carrot, tigernut flour, cassava flour, coconut flour, baking powder, cinnamon, maple syrup, coconut sugar, and coconut oil. Stir until combined. Add the gelatin egg and immediately combine into the mixture.

3. Use a soup spoon to scoop out 1½ tablespoons of the dough, then roll each scoop into a ball and place it on the baking sheet. Then lightly press down with your hand so it flattens into a disk.

4. Bake for 8 to 10 minutes, or until the tops start to turn golden brown. Cool on the baking sheet for at least 10 minutes before serving.

5. Store leftover cookies in an airtight container at room temperature for up to 5 days or in the refrigerator for up to 7 days.

Make it Easier: Make a double batch of cookie dough and freeze the uncooked dough in an airtight container for up to 3 months. Whenever you want a fresh, hot cookie, simply defrost the dough at room temperature for 1 hour, scoop the dough onto a baking sheet, and bake.

Per Serving: Calories: 88; Total Fat: 5g; Total Carbs: 10g; Fiber: 2g; Net Carbs: 8g; Protein: 1g

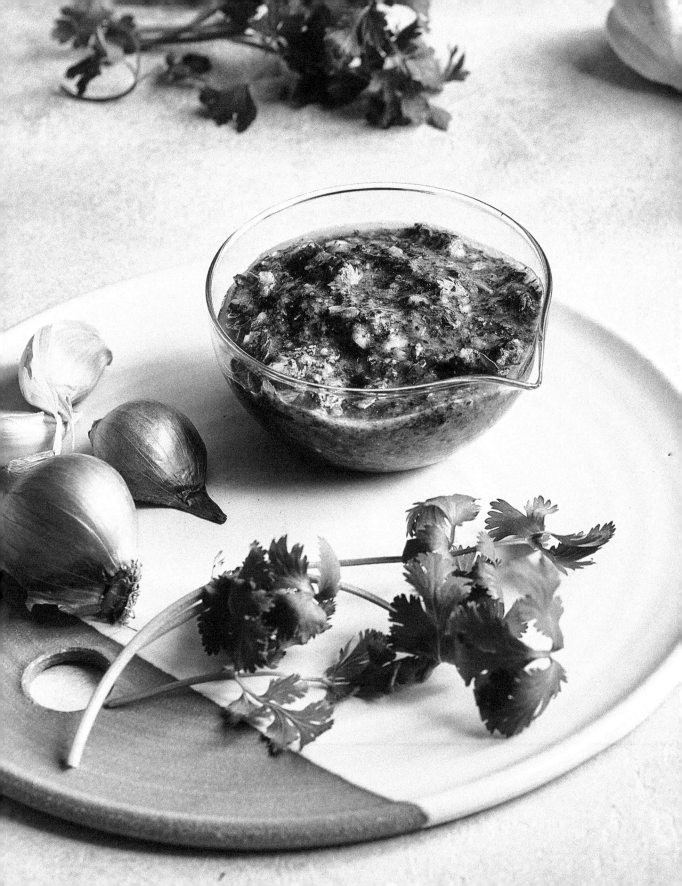

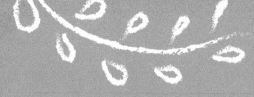

CHAPTER 10

STAPLES AND BASES

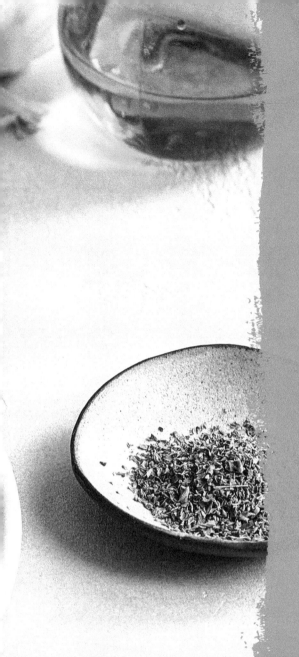

Chimichurri *page 182*

Coconut Milk

We are obsessed with coconut milk and it is perfect for the AIP way of eating. While the full-fat version in a can works great, the taste doesn't even come close to homemade coconut milk. There is just something better about the flavor and creaminess when it's freshly made. This is our favorite way to make it.

4 cups filtered water

2 cups unsweetened shredded coconut

1. In a large saucepan, heat the filtered water over medium heat. When it starts to simmer, remove from the heat. You don't want to use boiling water. Add the shredded coconut to the water. Infuse for 1 to 2 hours.

2. Pour the mixture into a blender. Blend on the highest speed for about 1 minute, or until fully combined.

3. Strain through a nut milk bag or cheesecloth and squeeze out all the liquid.

4. Pour into an airtight container and store in the refrigerator for up to 3 to 4 days.

Ingredient Spotlight: The fat in the coconut milk will separate from the water while it is in the refrigerator because there are no preservatives or fillers. Just shake or stir the coconut milk to combine before using. You may need to warm it up slightly to do this.

Per Serving (1 cup): Calories: 40; Total Fat: 4g; Total Carbs: 1g; Fiber: 0g; Net Carbs: 1g; Protein: 0g

Coconut Whipped Cream

This whipped cream is so easy to make and so delicious that you will want to eat it straight from the bowl. We recommend that you chill the bowl and the electric mixer beaters in the freezer for at least an hour before making this.

1 cup coconut cream, refrigerated overnight

2 tablespoons raw honey

1. In a medium bowl, use an electric mixer to beat together the coconut cream and honey for 5 to 10 minutes, or until fluffy.

2. Serve immediately, or store in an airtight container in the refrigerator for up to 5 days.

Swap or Substitute: If you don't have coconut cream, simply skim the solid white cream that rises to the top of a can of full-fat unsweetened coconut milk that has been refrigerated overnight.

Per Serving (2 tablespoons): Calories: 57; Total Fat: 5g; Total Carbs: 3g; Fiber: 0g; Net Carbs: 3g; Protein: 1g

Balsamic Vinaigrette

This recipe is super quick, super easy, and works great with any salad. We love pairing it with peppery arugula, as in our Apple Harvest Chicken Salad (page 99) and our Pan-Seared Filet Mignon with Arugula Salad (page 152). Make a batch on the weekend and it will last you all week.

¼ cup balsamic vinegar

4 teaspoons pure maple syrup

½ cup extra-virgin olive oil

Pinch pink Himalayan salt or sea salt

1. Pour the vinegar and maple syrup into a small bowl. Stirring constantly with a fork or small whisk, slowly add the olive oil in a small, steady stream until incorporated. Season with salt.

2. Store in an airtight container in the refrigerator for up to 7 days.

Ingredient Spotlight: Separation is natural when this dressing is stored in the refrigerator. Before serving all you need to do is shake it vigorously.

Per Serving (2 tablespoons): Calories: 165; Total Fat: 14g; Total Carbs: 4g; Fiber: 0g; Net Carbs: 4g; Protein: 0g

Cilantro Lime Vinaigrette

MAKES 2 CUPS / PREP TIME: 7 MINUTES

Cilantro and lime both have bright, fresh flavors that can wake up an ordinary dish. This is five-ingredient dressing is featured in many recipes in this book, including our Lime Shrimp Kebabs over Mixed Greens (page 119), Grilled Chimichurri Shrimp and Cucumber Mint Salad (page 120), and Cilantro Lime Shrimp and Avocado Salad (page 101).

2 cups fresh cilantro

½ cup lime juice

1 tablespoon red wine vinegar

1 garlic clove

½ cup extra-virgin olive oil

1. Place the cilantro, lime juice, vinegar, and garlic in a food processor or blender, and process to combine. Slowly pour in the olive oil in a steady stream and pulse until smooth.

2. Store in an airtight container in the refrigerator for up to 3 to 4 days.

Swap or Substitute: You can use white wine vinegar instead and swap avocado oil for extra-virgin olive oil, if you prefer.

Per Serving (2 tablespoons): Calories: 62; Total Fat: 7g; Total Carbs: 1g; Fiber: 0g; Net Carbs: 1g; Protein: 0g

Classic Ranch Dressing

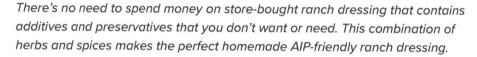

MAKES 1½ CUPS / PREP TIME: 10 MINUTES

There's no need to spend money on store-bought ranch dressing that contains additives and preservatives that you don't want or need. This combination of herbs and spices makes the perfect homemade AIP-friendly ranch dressing.

1 cup full-fat unsweetened coconut milk (store-bought or homemade, page 174)

1½ tablespoons apple cider vinegar

3 teaspoons onion powder

1 teaspoon garlic powder

1 teaspoon pink Himalayan salt or sea salt

1 tablespoon dried parsley or ¼ cup roughly chopped fresh parsley

¼ teaspoon dried dill or ½ teaspoon chopped fresh dill

1. Combine the coconut milk, vinegar, onion powder, garlic powder, salt, parsley, and dill in a blender and process until smooth.

2. Serve immediately, or store in an airtight container in the refrigerator for up to 7 days.

Swap or Substitute: Feel free to adjust the seasonings to your liking.

Per Serving (2 tablespoons): Calories: 41; Total Fat: 4g; Total Carbs: 1g; Fiber: 0g; Net Carbs: 1g; Protein: 1g

AIP Mayo

Traditional mayonnaise is egg-based. Since eggs are not part of the autoimmune protocol, our version uses palm shortening to provide the same texture. The mayo will continue to thicken in the refrigerator. It's AIP magic!

1 cup avocado oil

½ cup palm shortening

1 tablespoon lemon juice

¾ teaspoon pink Himalayan salt or sea salt

¾ teaspoon garlic powder

1. Combine the oil, shortening, lemon juice, salt, and garlic powder in a blender and process until smooth, about 3 minutes.

2. Store in an airtight container in the refrigerator for up to 7 days.

Ingredient Spotlight: Palm shortening is palm oil with some of the unsaturated fats removed, leaving it thick and creamy. If your grocery store doesn't carry it, you can find it in health food stores and online.

Per Serving (1 tablespoon): Calories: 178; Total Fat: 20g; Total Carbs: 0g; Fiber: 0g; Net Carbs: 0g; Protein: 0g

Garlic-Infused Oil

MAKES 1 CUP / PREP TIME: 5 MINUTES
COOK TIME: 30 MINUTES / INFUSION TIME: 2 HOURS

We love infusing oils to add an extra dimension of flavor. We are using extra-virgin olive oil in this version, so it's key to heat the oil at a low heat so that it doesn't oxidize and take on a rancid flavor. We have found the best temperature for infusing extra-virgin olive oil is 225°F, but just keep an eye on it to make sure it's at a very low simmer and you'll be fine.

1 cup extra-virgin olive oil

4 garlic cloves, peeled and cut in half

1. In a small saucepan, combine the olive oil and garlic and heat over low heat. Gently simmer for 30 minutes, making sure it doesn't begin to boil. Keep the heat on low.

2. Pour the mixture into a glass container with a lid. Let it sit, covered, at room temperature for 2 hours.

3. Use a slotted spoon to remove the garlic. Store the infused oil in the refrigerator for up to 3 to 4 days.

Ingredient Spotlight: The olive oil will solidify in the refrigerator. Let it come to room temperature, or run the sealed container under warm water to liquify.

Per Serving (1 tablespoon): Calories: 120; Total Fat: 14g; Total Carbs: 0g; Fiber: 0g; Net Carbs: 0g; Protein: 0g

Basil-Olive Pesto

Pesto is a versatile sauce that you can drizzle over seafood, AIP-friendly pasta, and vegetables. Traditional pesto is made with pine nuts and Parmesan cheese. Our fresh and flavorful version replaces these ingredients with kalamata olives, so this recipe fits even within the AIP-elimination phase.

2 cups packed fresh basil

¼ cup kalamata olives, pitted

4 garlic cloves

½ teaspoon pink Himalayan salt or sea salt

⅔ cup extra-virgin olive oil

1. Put the basil, olives, garlic, and salt in a food processor or blender. Process to combine.

2. Slowly pour in the olive oil and pulse until smooth.

3. Store in an airtight container in the refrigerator for up to 7 days.

Make It Easier: Double or triple this recipe and freeze any extra pesto in an ice cube tray. Transfer the frozen pesto cubes to an airtight container and store in the freezer for up to 1 month, and thaw a cube or two as you need them.

Per Serving (1 tablespoon): Calories: 84; Total Fat: 9g; Total Carbs: 0g; Fiber: 0g; Net Carbs: 0g; Protein: 0g

Chimichurri

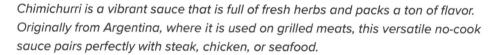

MAKES 1 CUP / PREP TIME: 5 MINUTES

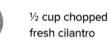

Chimichurri is a vibrant sauce that is full of fresh herbs and packs a ton of flavor. Originally from Argentina, where it is used on grilled meats, this versatile no-cook sauce pairs perfectly with steak, chicken, or seafood.

1 cup chopped
fresh parsley

½ cup chopped
fresh cilantro

1 medium shallot, diced

4 cloves garlic, minced

1 teaspoon pink Himalayan
salt or sea salt

1½ teaspoons
dried oregano

¼ cup red wine vinegar

½ cup extra-virgin olive oil

1. Put the parsley, cilantro, shallot, garlic, salt, oregano, and vinegar in a food processor or blender. Process to combine.

2. Slowly pour in the olive oil and pulse. Try not to blend the sauce until it's totally smooth—you want it to be slightly chunky.

3. Store in an airtight container in the refrigerator for up to 7 days.

Swap or Substitute: Traditional chimichurri sauce is made with just parsley, so feel free to use 1½ cups parsley and no cilantro, if you prefer.

Per Serving (2 tablespoons): Calories: 127; Total Fat: 14g; Total Carbs: 1g; Fiber: 0g; Net Carbs: 1g; Protein: 0g

Ginger Dipping Sauce

This sauce is a perfect way to add an East Asian–inspired burst of flavor, and you can use it in a variety of ways. Serve it as a dipping sauce with Oven-Fried Chicken Nuggets (page 64), use it to stir-fry vegetables, or drizzle it over our Shrimp Fried Rice (page 117). Don't be scared of the fish sauce; it provides incredible umami flavor. Our favorite brand is Red Boat.

½ cup coconut aminos

2 tablespoons raw honey

1 tablespoon white wine vinegar

1 teaspoon grated fresh ginger

1 garlic clove, minced

2 teaspoons fish sauce

1. In a small saucepan over medium-low heat, combine the coconut aminos, honey, vinegar, ginger, garlic, and fish sauce.

2. Whisk the mixture together and cook for 10 minutes, or until the sauce has thickened.

3. Store in an airtight container in the refrigerator for up to 7 days.

Ingredient Spotlight: Using coconut aminos is a wonderful way to achieve depth of flavor. It's a great substitute for soy sauce and does not contain gluten, which makes it perfect for AIP recipes.

Per Serving (2 tablespoons): Calories: 28; Total Fat: 0g; Total Carbs: 6g; Fiber: 0g; Net Carbs: 6g; Protein: 2g

"Nomato" Sauce

This is our take on tomato sauce—except with no tomatoes. We love using this in any Italian-style dish. Make sure to taste the sauce and adjust the seasonings to your liking. If you have one, an immersion blender will make this dish even easier—just blend it right in the pot. And if you prefer a thinner sauce, just add more filtered water.

1 tablespoon avocado oil

1 yellow onion, diced

4 garlic cloves, minced

½ pound carrots, chopped

1 red beet, chopped

½ cup filtered water

1 tablespoon lemon juice

1 teaspoon dried oregano

Pinch pink Himalayan salt or sea salt

1. Heat the avocado oil in a large saucepan over medium-high heat, and add the onion and garlic. Sauté, stirring constantly, until softened, about 5 minutes. Add the carrots, beet, and water, and bring the mixture to a boil. Reduce the heat to low, cover, and simmer for 30 minutes, or until the carrots and beets are fork-tender.

2. Carefully transfer the mixture to a blender, add the lemon juice and oregano, and season with salt. Blend until smooth. The liquid will be hot, so place a dish towel over the top of the blender before turning it on.

3. Serve immediately, or store in an airtight container in the refrigerator for up to 7 days or in the freezer for 3 months.

Swap or Substitute: If you are a garlic lover like us, use even more cloves. We also love adding fresh basil to this sauce.

Per Serving (1 cup): Calories: 106; Total Fat: 6g; Total Carbs: 15g; Fiber: 4g; Net Carbs: 11g; Protein: 2g

"Cheese" Sauce

MAKES 4 CUPS / PREP TIME: 10 MINUTES / COOK TIME: 10 MINUTES

This sauce is extremely versatile and has the look, texture, and taste of cheese. We love to use it in our "Cheesy" Chicken and Broccoli Casserole (page 130). The secret in this recipe is the bacon fat. Just make sure to check the ingredients on the bacon package and ensure any added spices are AIP-friendly.

1 head cauliflower, chopped into large florets (about 4 cups)

4 garlic cloves

1 cup full-fat unsweetened coconut milk (store-bought or homemade, page 174)

½ cup chicken bone broth (store-bought or homemade, page 190)

¼ cup bacon fat

1 tablespoon fish sauce

1 tablespoon apple cider vinegar

Pinch pink Himalayan salt or sea salt

1. In a large pot filled with 1 inch of filtered water, insert a steamer basket and put the cauliflower florets in the steamer. Cover and bring the water to a boil. Steam the cauliflower for 10 minutes, or until tender.

2. Combine the steamed cauliflower, garlic, coconut milk, bone broth, bacon fat, fish sauce, vinegar, and salt in a food processor or blender. Process for about 5 minutes, or until a smooth sauce forms.

3. Pour the finished sauce into an airtight container and store in the refrigerator for up to 3 to 4 days.

Ingredient Spotlight: To render bacon fat, cook at least 4 slices of bacon in a skillet or cast-iron pan over medium-high heat (as in our Open-Face Breakfast Sandwich, page 83). When the bacon is cooked, remove the slices from the pan. Strain the fat into a jar and store it in the refrigerator for up to 1 month.

Per Serving (¼ cup): Calories: 68; Total Fat: 6g; Total Carbs: 3g; Fiber: 1g; Net Carbs: 2g; Protein: 1g

AIP Barbecue Sauce

MAKES 4 CUPS / PREP TIME: 10 MINUTES / COOK TIME: 30 MINUTES

This AIP-friendly barbecue sauce contains no nightshades, seeds, or refined sugars. Despite not using any of these traditional barbecue sauce ingredients in this recipe, it looks and tastes just like the barbecue sauce you are used to eating. If you have an immersion blender, puree the sauce right in the pot to make it even easier. Make a big batch so you always have it on hand.

4 carrots, peeled and cut into 1-inch pieces

2 apples, peeled, cored, and cut into large chunks

2 cups blackberries

1 yellow onion, peeled and cut into chunks

¼ cup blackstrap molasses

¾ cup apple cider vinegar

4 teaspoons garlic powder

4 teaspoons onion powder

3 teaspoons liquid smoke

3 teaspoons pink Himalayan salt or sea salt

2 teaspoons ground ginger

¼ cup filtered water

6 tablespoons pure maple syrup

1. In a medium-large pot over medium heat, combine the carrots, apples, blackberries, onion, molasses, apple cider vinegar, garlic powder, onion powder, liquid smoke, salt, ginger, and water. Simmer, covered, for 30 minutes. Stir in the maple syrup.

2. Working in batches, carefully transfer the mixture to a blender and puree. Be extremely careful not to fill the blender too full of the hot mixture, and cover the lid with a dish towel while blending.

3. Store in an airtight container in the refrigerator for up to 2 months.

Ingredient Spotlight: Liquid smoke is made from condensing the smoke of burning wood. You can find bottled liquid smoke at your local grocery store in the condiment aisle.

Per Serving (2 tablespoons): Calories: 40; Total Fat: 0g; Total Carbs: 10g; Fiber: 1g; Net Carbs: 9g; Protein: 0g

Gelatin Egg

Gelatin eggs are the perfect solution for AIP baking! We use them in biscuits, muffins, waffles, and even desserts. Use these as a one-to-one egg substitute in any baking recipe that you are trying to make AIP-friendly.

¼ cup filtered water

1 tablespoon beef gelatin powder

1. Pour the water into a small saucepan and sprinkle the gelatin on top. Let it sit for 3 minutes, or until the mixture hardens.

2. Place the saucepan on the stove over low heat. Allow the mixture to melt for 1 to 2 minutes. Then use a handheld electric mixer or a whisk to mix until it becomes frothy.

3. Use the prepared gelatin egg immediately.

Ingredient Spotlight: The gelatin egg will harden soon after it's prepared, so it's important to use in your recipe immediately after you make it.

Per Serving: Calories: 10; Total Fat: 0g; Total Carbs: 2g; Fiber: 0g; Net Carbs: 2g; Protein: 0g

Shredded Chicken

You will always find shredded chicken in our refrigerators. It's easy to make a batch on the weekend and then use it all week in salads, casseroles, stir-fries, and soups. It's almost as easy as the rotisserie chicken you buy at the supermarket, but a lot less expensive—plus, you know exactly what's in it.

4 boneless, skinless chicken thighs

1. Put the chicken thighs in a medium saucepan and add just enough filtered water to cover completely. Cover the pan and bring to a simmer over medium heat.

2. As soon as the water reaches a simmer, reduce the heat to low and cook the chicken for 10 to 15 minutes, or until it's fully cooked through.

3. Remove the chicken thighs from the water and let cool before shredding with two forks.

4. Serve immediately, or store in an airtight container in the refrigerator for up to 3 to 4 days or in the freezer for 3 months.

Swap or Substitute: We like to use chicken thighs in this recipe because they have a higher fat content and more flavor. But use boneless, skinless chicken breasts if you prefer.

Per Serving: Calories: 234; Total Fat: 7g; Total Carbs: 0g; Fiber: 0g; Net Carbs: 0g; Protein: 38g

Cauliflower Mash Three Ways

SERVES 4 / PREP TIME: 5 MINUTES / COOK TIME: 15 MINUTES

Cauliflower is so versatile and makes a terrific AIP-friendly substitute for mashed potatoes. The basic version tastes terrific, but we also provided you with our two favorite variations. Look for precut cauliflower florets at the grocery store to make this recipe even quicker. And if you don't feel like taking out an appliance, you can mash this all in a big bowl using a handheld potato masher.

BASIC MASH

1 head cauliflower, cut into florets

3 tablespoons extra-virgin olive oil

1 teaspoon garlic powder

1 teaspoon pink Himalayan salt or sea salt

RANCH VERSION

¼ cup Classic Ranch Dressing (page 178)

HORSERADISH VERSION

1 tablespoon prepared horseradish

Ingredient Spotlight: You can find prepared horseradish in the refrigerated section of grocery stores. The only ingredients should be horseradish, vinegar, and salt.

1. Set a steamer basket in a large pot and add enough filtered water to fill the pot just below the basket. Put the cauliflower florets in the steamer basket. Cover and bring to a boil. Steam for 10 minutes, or until tender.

2. Transfer the steamed cauliflower to a food processor or blender and add the olive oil and garlic powder. Process for 2 minutes, or until smooth.

3. Season with salt, and mix in any extras you desire.

4. Serve immediately, or store in an airtight container in the refrigerator for up to 5 days.

Per Serving (Basic): Calories: 129; Total Fat: 11g; Total Carbs: 8g; Fiber: 3g; Net Carbs: 5g; Protein: 3g

Per Serving (Ranch): Calories: 149; Total Fat: 13g; Total Carbs: 8g; Fiber: 3g; Net Carbs: 5g; Protein: 3g

Per Serving (Horseradish): Calories: 136; Total Fat: 11g; Total Carbs: 8g; Fiber: 3g; Net Carbs: 7g; Protein: 3g

Chicken Bone Broth

SERVES 12 / PREP TIME: 5 MINUTES / COOK TIME: 11 TO 27 HOURS

The healing benefits of bone broth are numerous and include improved diges-tion and immunity health. We recommend drinking a cup a day as part of your healing journey. The long cooking time enables you to extract the highest level of nutrients possible from the bones. If you can find them, use chicken feet, necks, and backs, as these have more gelatin. You can sometimes get these from the butcher or the meat counter at the supermarket.

2 to 3 pounds raw chicken bones

1⅓ cups roughly chopped onion

1⅓ cups roughly chopped celery

1⅓ cups roughly chopped carrots

1 tablespoon apple cider vinegar

2 bay leaves

1 teaspoon pink Himalayan salt or sea salt

About 16 cups filtered water

1. Preheat the oven to 350°F.

2. Place the chicken bones in a large roasting pan and roast for 30 minutes.

3. Transfer the bones to a slow cooker and add the other ingredients. Be careful not to overfill your slow cooker—less water is okay.

4. Cover and cook on low for 18 to 24 hours.

5. Cool the broth for about 20 minutes, then use a strainer to carefully remove the bones and vegeta-bles. Discard them.

6. Store the broth in an airtight container in the refrigerator for up to 3 to 4 days or in the freezer for up to 6 months.

Make it Easier: If you don't have a slow cooker, put the roasted bones in a large pot along with all the other ingredients. Fill the pot with enough filtered water to cover the bones by about 1 inch. Bring the broth to a boil, then reduce the heat to a simmer and cover. After 2 hours, use a slotted spoon to skim off any impurities that floated to the surface and discard. Continue to cook the broth on the lowest heat for 8 to 24 hours. Make sure it isn't cooking at too high of a temperature or it may become cloudy; if it does, it's still fine to drink.

Per Serving (1 cup): Calories: 45; Total Fat: 0g; Total Carbs: 1g; Fiber: 0g; Net Carbs: 1g; Protein: 10g

Beef Bone Broth

SERVES 12 / PREP TIME: 5 MINUTES / COOK TIME: 11 TO 27 HOURS

Beef bone broth is a staple in our kitchens and is used as the base of many of our soups. It is gut-healing, nourishing, and has a rich, incredible depth of flavor. Look for high-quality bones from grass-fed cattle, which you can get from the butcher or the meat counter at your supermarket. To make a broth with the most collagen, try to use feet, knuckles, necks, and backs.

2 to 3 pounds raw beef bones

1⅓ cups roughly chopped onion

1⅓ cups roughly chopped celery

1⅓ cups roughly chopped carrots

1 tablespoon apple cider vinegar

2 bay leaves

1 teaspoon pink Himalayan salt or sea salt

About 16 cups filtered water

1. Preheat the oven to 350°F.

2. Put the beef bones in a large roasting pan and roast for 30 minutes.

3. Transfer the bones to a slow cooker and add the onion, celery, carrots, apple cider vinegar, bay leaves, salt, and water. Be careful not to overfill your slow cooker—less water is okay.

4. Cover and cook on low for 18 to 24 hours.

5. Cool the broth for about 20 minutes, then use a strainer to carefully remove the bones and vegetables. Discard them.

6. Store the broth in an airtight container in the refrigerator for up to 3 to 4 days or in the freezer for up to 6 months.

Make it Easier: If you don't have a slow cooker, put the roasted bones in a large pot along with all the other ingredients. Fill the pot with enough filtered water so the bones are covered by about 1 inch. Bring the broth to a boil, then reduce the heat to a simmer and cover. After 2 hours, use a slotted spoon to skim off any impurities that floated to the surface and discard. Continue to cook the broth on the lowest heat for 8 to 24 hours. Make sure it isn't cooking at too high of a temperature or it may become cloudy; if it does, it's still fine to drink.

Per Serving (1 cup): Calories: 40; Total Fat: 0g; Total Carbs: 0g; Fiber: 0g; Net Carbs: 0g; Protein: 10g

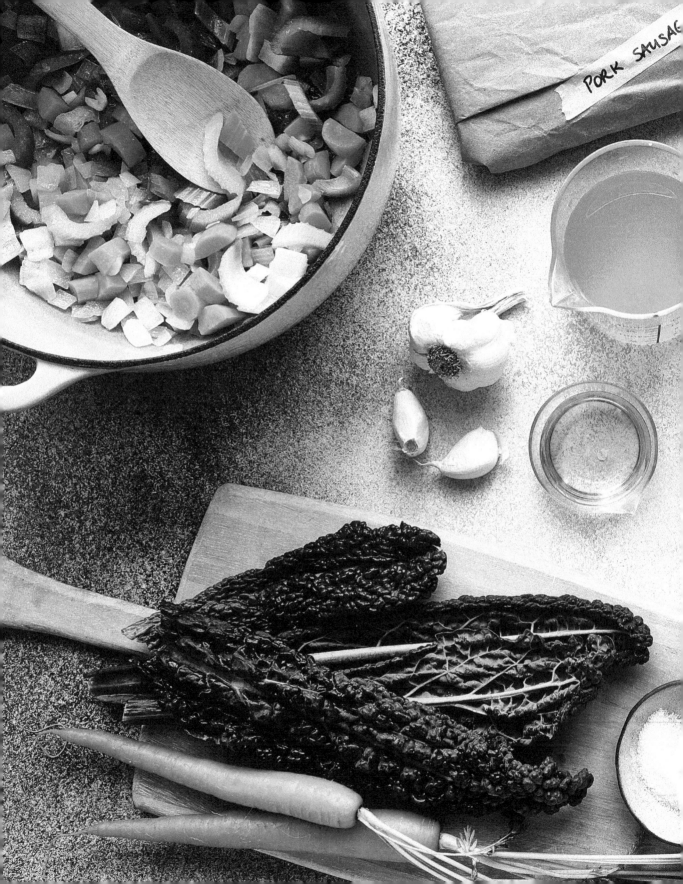

MEASUREMENT CONVERSIONS

VOLUME EQUIVALENTS (LIQUID)

US Standard	US Standard (ounces)	Metric (approx.)
2 tablespoons	1 fl. oz.	30 mL
¼ cup	2 fl. oz.	60 mL
½ cup	4 fl. oz.	120 mL
1 cup	8 fl. oz.	240 mL
1½ cups	12 fl. oz.	355 mL
2 cups or 1 pint	16 fl. oz.	475 mL
4 cups or 1 quart	32 fl. oz.	1 L
1 gallon	128 fl. oz.	4 L

OVEN TEMPERATURES

Fahrenheit (F)	Celsius (C) (approx.)
250°F	120°C
300°F	150°C
325°F	165°C
350°F	180°C
375°F	190°C
400°F	200°C
425°F	220°C
450°F	230°C

VOLUME EQUIVALENTS (DRY)

US Standard	Metric (approx.)
⅛ teaspoon	0.5 mL
¼ teaspoon	1 mL
½ teaspoon	2 mL
¾ teaspoon	4 mL
1 teaspoon	5 mL
1 tablespoon	15 mL
¼ cup	59 mL
⅓ cup	79 mL
½ cup	118 mL
⅔ cup	156 mL
¾ cup	177 mL
1 cup	235 mL
2 cups or 1 pint	475 mL
3 cups	700 mL
4 cups or 1 quart	1 L

WEIGHT EQUIVALENTS

US Standard	Metric (approx.)
½ ounce	15 g
1 ounce	30 g
2 ounces	60 g
4 ounces	115 g
8 ounces	225 g
12 ounces	340 g
16 ounces or 1 pound	455 g

RESOURCES

CleanKetoLifestyle.com

Head over to our website for more recipes and resources. We also offer group programs and one-on-one coaching to help people implement the autoimmune protocol.

The Autoimmune Keto Cookbook **by Karissa Long and Katie Austin** (Rockridge Press, 2019)

This book, also written by Karissa and Katie, includes 85 keto recipes, five weeks of meal plans, exercise routines, and specific advice on how to eat a ketogenic diet when you are out in social situations.

The Paleo Approach: Reverse Autoimmune Disease and Heal Your Body **by Sarah D. Ballantyne, PhD** (Victory Belt Publishing, 2014)

Dr. Ballantyne breaks down the science and medical research on autoimmune disease and diet, and explains why you should follow the autoimmune protocol if you have an autoimmune disease.

OUR FAVORITE
AIP-FRIENDLY BRANDS

Arrowroot starch: Bob's Red Mill

Barbecue sauce: KC Natural Mastodon

Beef gelatin: Great Lakes, Vital Proteins

Bone broth: Bonafide Provisions, Kettle & Fire

Cassava flour: Otto's Natural, Anthony's

Coconut aminos: Coconut Secret

Coconut cream: Native Forest, Trader Joe's, Thrive Market

Coconut flour: Bob's Red Mill

Coconut milk: Native Forest Simple, Trader Joe's, Thrive Market

Coconut sugar: Nutiva, Thrive Market

Coconut yogurt: Anita's, GT's CocoYo

Collagen peptides powder: Vital Proteins

Fish sauce: Red Boat

Lard: Fatworks, Epic

MCT oil: Nutiva, Viva Naturals

Plantain chips: Banana Organic, Terra

Pork rinds: Epic, 4505 Meats

Shirataki noodles and rice: Miracle Noodles

Spice blends: Primal Palate AIP line

Tignernut flour: Organic Gemini

Vanilla powder: Terrasoul Superfoods

INDEX